Logic
of
Operating Room
Nursing
Third Edition

Jacqueline Willingham Cordner
RN, CNOR

Operating Room Consultant

Medical Economics Books
Oradell, New Jersey 07649

Library of Congress Cataloging in Publication Data

Cordner, Jacqueline Willingham.
    Logic of operating room nursing.

    1. Operating room nursing. I. Title. [DNLM:
1. Surgical nursing. WY 161 C795L]
RD99.C72   1984   610.73'677   83-20385
ISBN 0-87489-359-3

Design by *A Good Thing Inc.*

ISBN 0-87489-359-3

Medical Economics Company Inc.
Oradell, New Jersey 07649·

Printed in the United States of America

Table of Contents

Foreword

Sound judgment and appropriate decision making are the essence of professional practice. Logical thinking, based on sound principles of the natural and behavioral sciences, must precede any action taken in the care of surgical patients. Each patient entrusted to the care of the operating room team has the right to expect thoughtful, considerate, and reasonable care. Each member of the team is responsible for his or her own actions in rendering this care.

Jacqueline Willingham Cordner has devoted her professional nursing career to caring for and sharing with others. As an operating room staff nurse she cared for patients by sharing her knowledge and skills as a direct patient care team member. As an operating room nursing administrator, she cared about the development of the members of her staff—the nurses, surgical technologists, and nursing assistants. She afforded them the opportunity to grow and develop personally and professionally/vocationally. Through her writings and public speaking, she has shared her knowledge and dedication to OR nursing with her colleagues.

This third edition of *Logic of Operating Room Nursing*, like the previous editions, provides useful tools for making sound judgments related to patient care in the OR. The chapter on attitudes emphasizes personal morals, values, and ethics essential to a surgical conscience that is always aware, always knows right from wrong, and always responds appropriately. "The Mental Lineup" and "The Four-Clue System" offer logical methods of thinking before acting to solve the inevitable problems faced daily in the OR. Every patient and every operation is different. Therefore, as emphasized in the last chapter, patient care must be individualized. Some of the technical procedural components inherent in OR nursing, of necessity, are outlined to create awareness of and concern for the safety and welfare of every patient.

Although the pronoun she/her is used to refer to the nurse and he/his to the patient, surgeon, and anesthesiologist, it must be acknowledged that gender is irrelevant to genuine concern for people, be they patients or colleagues. Teamwork focuses on the unique human being we call patient who needs the expertise and efficiency of knowledgeable people to care for him or her in the OR. That is the logic of OR nursing.

Lucy Jo Atkinson, R.N., M.S.

Publisher's Notes

Jacqueline Willingham Cordner, R.N., C.N.O.R., who currently serves the nursing profession as operating room consultant, is former Director of the Operating Room and Recovery Room at Riverside General Hospital in Secaucus, New Jersey, where she was instrumental in designing and instituting the modern systems now in use at that institution. Prior to her work there, she served for almost 20 years as Director of the Operating Room and Post Anesthesia Room at Hackensack (N.J.) Medical Center (formerly Hackensack Hospital). She received her diploma in professional nursing from the Roosevelt Hospital School of Nursing in New York, and the degree of Bachelor of Arts cum laude from Jersey City State College.

Among her many contributions to medical publishing, Mrs. Cordner wrote *Manual of Operating Room Management* (Medical Economics Books), two previous editions of *Logic of Operating Room Nursing* (Springer), and coauthored *Doodle Dictionary for the O.R.* (Bard-Parker). She was guest columnist for *O.R. Reporter* (Davis & Geck), and wrote the script of a motion picture, *Positioning the Patient for Surgery—Principles and Practices* (AORN National Film Committee).

Her journalistic achievements include two award-winning articles for the *AORN Journal* and several contributions to *RN*, on which she served as an editorial board member from 1959-1973. In addition, she has presented many public addresses, and has initiated and conducted several educational programs and seminars for the nursing community.

Mrs. Cordner served as president of AORN of New Jersey, Chapter 1, from 1968-1971. She has been a panel member at annual meetings of the national AORN, chairman of the national organization's Audio-Visual Committee, and charter member of the AORN-AORT Advisory Board.

Through her various activities as writer, speaker, and nursing administrator, Jacqueline Cordner has sought to educate nurses and technologists in the principles and practice of OR nursing, always with emphasis on the importance of knowing what you are doing. As she puts it, "If you understand the principles of OR nursing, you're equipped to practice anywhere."

Lucy Jo Atkinson, R.N., M.S., who wrote the Foreword, is Director of Educational Services at Ethicon, Inc., Somerville, New Jersey, and editor of *Point of View* magazine. She was previously Operating Room Supervisor at Children's Hospital of Pittsburgh and Assistant Director of Nursing Service in charge of Operating Rooms and Recovery Rooms at Cedars of Lebanon Hospital in Los Angeles.

Miss Atkinson was a member of the Editorial Committee of the *AORN Journal,* and wrote many articles for that and other nursing publications. She is coauthor of *Berry & Kohn's Introduction to Operating Room Technique* (McGraw-Hill) and lectures to many nursing and technologist groups in the United States and abroad.

Acknowledgments

I am most grateful to my husband, Harold J. Cordner, M.D., attending anesthesiologist, Hackensack Medical Center, Hackensack, New Jersey, for his encouragement and invaluable assistance while I prepared this book, and to our children for their patience.

Also, thinking back, I owe a debt of gratitude to Edythe L. Alexander, original author of *Alexander's Care of the Patient in Surgery,* who not only taught me operating room nursing years ago, but who fostered within me the desire for excellence in the performance and management of operating room nursing.

Introduction

Competent professional nurses are needed as health team members for the care of the patient in the operating room. It is obvious that resources for their education should be available. Consequently, *Logic of Operating Room Nursing*—a basic OR educational tool—has been revised and updated from its two former editions, which were used extensively in the past. It is designed for the new staff member, as well as for the "not-so-new" operating room nurse.

Today, the operating room nurse is an organized meld of knowledge—patient-care oriented; technique oriented; task oriented; and scientifically oriented. She sees that the principles of science, medicine, and nursing are practiced, and the challenge of continual rapid advancements in medical techniques and instrumentation keeps her from stagnation.

A new nurse entering the specialty of OR nursing is eager to learn, but is overwhelmed by the techniques and applicable functions being taught. The cry "Will I ever learn?" can be turned around to "Now I understand!" by having the principles (basic background knowledge) behind the practice pointed out. An operating room nurse, even with a few years' experience, may not be functioning at her optimum, because a basic knowledge and logical pattern of thinking have not been instilled.

The purpose of this book is to equip the operating room nurse with the pertinent basics of OR nursing and to promote a logical pattern of thinking. This engenders personal satisfaction, completeness in work, and, consequently, optimum individualized care for each patient.

To be of benefit to operating room nurses in different kinds of hospitals, it was essential to make the book adaptable to any institution, regardless of bed capacity, location, available funds, surgical specialties, and operating room staff complement. The book does not encroach upon institutional policies or suggest changes in technique—e.g., it does not describe a particular sterile table arrangement or scrub procedure. Rather, it develops principles of operating room nursing that will correlate with different teaching programs and varied practices.

The subject has been treated from the individual nurse's view of the operating room situation and of the many functions she has to perform. The care and use of articles of surgery (instruments, sutures, drugs, etc.) are considered, along with the cardinal factors of positioning and draping the patient. Two chapters demonstrate and emphasize the thought process of the operating room nurse in actual surgery—how she can visualize and anticipate the transactions, and thereby become adept in preparing the setups and assisting at the operative field.

The responsibilities of the OR nurse to the patient on admission to the operating room suite, to the surgeon's preferences, and to the anesthesiologist are dealt with throughout the book. Hopefully, the chapter on individualizing patient care will serve as a constant reminder that each patient is different, and that individual needs must be recognized and met. Medicolegal documentation is also stressed.

In view of the fact that cesarean sections are now commonly performed in the delivery room, obstetrical nurses must also be equipped with operating room knowledge. This book offers them the proper background in aseptic techniques, instrumentation, and other elements applicable to the safe delivery of patient care and the maintenance of a safe environment.

Presented in outline form, the text is concise, and includes examples that serve to emphasize or explain the brief statements. Therefore, the operating room nurse can use the book for study and thus be better prepared for the instructional classes. It accelerates the OR learning process.

Learning can be defined as "gaining knowledge, comprehension, and skill." As you *read* this book, *think* about the subject matter; *visualize* the article, action, or situation; and *apply* the principles. Read—Think—Visualize—Apply.

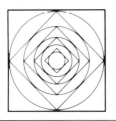

Chapter 1
The Surgical Team

A successful operation depends on the smooth, efficient performance of the surgical team. The team required for routine operative procedures varies in number—usually from four to seven people. The number increases for complex procedures such as open heart surgery; instances when sophisticated equipment is in use; and when the presence of a cardiologist, pathologist, or radiologist is indicated. The team normally referred to as the surgical team consists of:

ANESTHESIOLOGIST—the doctor who administers the anesthesia.

SURGEON (scrubbed)—the doctor who performs the surgery.

FIRST ASSISTANT (scrubbed)—the doctor who assists the surgeon with ligatures, support of part, etc.

SECOND ASSISTANT (scrubbed)—the doctor who usually holds the retractors.

SCRUB NURSE (or scrub assistant)—a nurse or surgical technologist who prepares the setup, and assists the surgeon by passing instruments, sutures, etc.

CIRCULATING NURSE—a professional registered nurse who is free to obtain supplies, answer the anesthesiologist's requests, deliver supplies to the sterile field, carry out the nursing care plan, etc.

There are times when a circulating nurse may require an assistant, e.g., when positioning a patient. Certain procedures do not require a second assistant doctor.

A dictionary meaning of *team* is "a number of persons associated in some joint action"—certainly appropriate to the operating room. And *teamwork* is defined as "work of a team with reference to coordination of effort and to collective efficiency." Each member of a surgical team assumes a responsibility for the patient. In surgery, a patient is entrusting himself wholly to our care. He is placed in a dependent position in which he has little or no control of the activities.

The qualities of an effective team are mutual trust, good communication between the members of the team, knowledge of procedures, and skill. Each member knows that all efforts are made for the benefit of the patient. The physician depends on the nursing team to provide the necessary instruments, equipment, and supplies, and he assumes that the team members know how to use them and care for them. In addition, he expects the team to be well-organized and confident. (The team can acquire this confidence, for example, by referring to the surgeon's preference cards, by studying written procedures, and by holding frequent in-service conferences.)

Remember, teamwork is a requisite for collective efficiency.

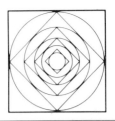

Chapter 2
Personal Attitude

The people you work with, and those you serve, evaluate you by your work and by your personal attitude. Personal attitude influences all aspects of hospital relationships—from a friendly morning greeting to the economy of hospital equipment.

PERSONAL APPEARANCE

Good posture, cleanliness, neatness—all are indications of a person's self-respect. If, in addition, a nurse is enthusiastic about life, her job, and herself, there is an aura of alertness about her that makes a tremendous impact upon the people she works with, and her performance as a team member rates high. These qualities are prerequisite for an operating room nurse.

Consider this: If a nurse does not like herself enough to exemplify pride in her personal appearance, no amount of supervision or criticism will stimulate her to develop that quality. Similarly, a lack of interest in personal appearance will express itself in lack of enthusiasm to work in an organized situation, to exercise care in setting up a case, and to carry out an assignment to its completion.

CONSIDERATION OF OTHERS

Surgical operations are carried out in team fashion (surgeon, assistant, scrub assistant, circulating nurse), and the need for harmony is paramount. Consideration of others is exemplified by tolerance, kindness, gentleness, and even the kind word and smile that is welcomed by everyone. No matter how skilled you may be, gentleness must be present. In comparison, arrogance breeds defensiveness in others and thus defeats group function.

COOPERATION

No matter how large or small the hospital is in which you are employed, cooperation is a *constant* process. You cooperate by teaching, that is, by passing on knowledge you have gained from a certain case or procedure. For example, if a surgeon desires a change in his routine or choice of suture, report it to your supervisor. You will use the system of communication set up in the department, whether it is a Kardex, procedure book, or daily conference manual. Cooperation has several effects:

1. The patient benefits, as better care is achieved.

2. The nursing staff benefits, by becoming more efficient and secure in their work.

3. Errors are not repeated, and time loss is avoided.

The OR department sets goals and objectives for the year, and must ready itself for the impact of advanced surgical procedures, system changes, and stringent cost-containment programs. A cooperative staff is essential for success. To become a cooperative member of the staff, you must:

1. Become aware of your educational needs.

2. Follow directions and enthusiastically try to make the new systems work.

3. Assure your criticisms are constructive.

4. Be willing to help attain department goals.

Cooperation is a give-and-take attitude that is a *sine qua non* for group function. There is no place for selfishness.

PROFESSIONAL CONDUCT

The surgeons and nurses you admire always maintain a professional attitude while at work, and thereby promote good rapport between co-workers. In surgery, where everyone is responsible for getting the job done, any social relationships become professional relationships. Friendships must stand up, and they will, when an individual values a friendship enough to grant the other person respect while performing his or her work.

Inappropriate forms of address, wise remarks, references to social activities, loud talk, or singing—all mean lack of concern for others, lack of sensitivity as to how such behavior might affect the people under tension at the time of an operation. The result is that proper relationships between doctor, nurse, and patient are destroyed.

Mature, professional conduct creates the opposite effect. People respect you; you attain more cooperation from your co-workers; and, above all, the patient feels more confident if the environment is a professional one at a time of great importance in his life. Patients have many preconceived concepts of hospitals, personnel, and surgery that may be magnified by conversation, noise, and observation of conduct. Many have been predisposed to information and misinformation by the dramatic media, and such influences have heightened the anxiety level.

Although the noise, surgical terminology, and conversation concerning patients' ills are everyday occurrences to the operating room nurse, they are strange to a patient, and he may misinterpret them. *For example:*

1. Laughter in the corridor becomes laughter about the patient.

2. A debate as to who is going to scrub, or an argument in the hallway, increases the patient's nervousness. No one wants to be operated upon under such disturbing conditions.

3. Words such as "knife" and "scissors," although commonplace to a nurse, send a scare into a patient.

4. A patient does not want to lose his identity as a person with a name. To be referred to as "the gallbladder" makes him feel lost and insecure.

EMOTIONS AND PERSONALITIES

During surgery, your personal feelings and responses toward people or circumstances must not show. Surgery is no time for an exhibition on your part—the patient comes first. Smart answers, sighs, and the like will gain no victory for you or the patient. They will not alter the situation or add to your reputation, but they will increase tension. *For example:*

1. Anger demonstrates a feeling of helplessness. Ask yourself: "Should this situation make me feel helpless?" If not, the anger is the other person's problem. So do not get involved; you will be emotionally free to work unencumbered.

2. Do not misinterpret tension for anger. A surgeon is under tension if he "yells" for a clamp, and continues to do so until you give him the correct one. Remember, he has to cope with an emergent situation, and it is natural that he respond sharply, with tenseness.

Refrain from unnecessary comment. Your poise will be maintained, and your ability will be evident. *For example:*

1. A comment is sometimes an attempt to get off the hook. To say "I didn't pick this set of instruments" or "Nobody tells me anything" means trying to place the blame elsewhere. To blame is a common phenomenon. Placing the blame on someone else doesn't help the situation. How to solve the problem at hand must be the only concern.

2. By maintaining poise and solving the problem, you create the proper situation. You send for the instruments the surgeon desires that are missing from the set. Instead of making a comment, you say to yourself: "I just learned something," or "Perhaps I should get more information on this procedure when the operation is over," or "Next time I will check my instrument setup before I begin."

The following are results of refraining from unnecessary comment:

1. The surgeon may apologize or explain his reactions.

2. The surgeon may be more willing and interested to teach you his preferences.

3. You will be better equipped, materially and mentally, for the next time.

4. You will demonstrate that your concern for the patient's needs supersedes your personal needs.

Remember, everyone in the operating room is under tension, not only you. You are an assistant. Forget yourself, drop resentment, and *think* about the other fellow.

What are the personalities of operating room nurses? Here are some:

- The "selfless" nurse—gives all, but inwardly expects a return.
- The "selfish" nurse—is after her own needs.
- The "anxious" nurse—is insecure.
- The "arrogant" nurse—seeks prestige.
- The "silly" nurse—is immature, seeks escape.
- The "defensive" nurse—feels others get a better deal.
- The "hostile" nurse—is angry at herself and the world.
- The "well-integrated" nurse—is well adjusted and secure.

Our personality makeups differ because of past experiences, ambitions or lack of ambitions, goals in life, feelings toward mankind, and the need to satisfy one's self. But any one of us may, at times, demonstrate one or another of those traits. Self-examination and an honest effort to overcome one's faults result in a happier person, and certainly a more efficient and desirable member of an operating room staff.

ATTITUDE TOWARD RESPONSIBILITY

Everyone desires responsibility, for it is indicative of the trust of others, and it encourages action. If you are given responsibility, remember that it is not something you pick up today and discard tomorrow. *For example:*

1. Proper identification of a patient is of prime importance. You are trusted to recheck the patient's identity when he enters the operating room. No matter how many tasks demand your attention, you must re-identify the patient. Do you *always* do that?

2. When you are responsible for supplying a room correctly, do you observe the small items? Do you report the depletion of certain supplies, or a cabinet door that does not close correctly? That would be fulfilling your "unassigned" responsibility as well as your assigned task.

3. Do you clean equipment after use? Do you return it to its proper location? Do you assess its completeness and readiness for the next person?

CONSCIENCE TOWARD TECHNIQUE

You have a very responsible position. Every setup a doctor uses is prepared by a nurse. A good part of the doctor's success and the patient's well-being is in your hands. Remember that obligation. Only you can answer the question "Did I use good surgical technique while preparing for and executing this procedure?" Everyone connected with the procedure is sure you did. Have you betrayed those people and yourself?

Sterility is a matter of either. . . or. Articles are either sterile or unsterile. There is no "almost sterile." When any question about sterility arises, consider the article unsterile. *For example:*

1. An area is draped for a fractured hip. You did the draping and are satisfied with the technique. The first assistant may question the sterility of one sheet. Have that sheet removed, or the entire drape, if necessary. Debate is absurd.

2. You open a "peel-away" packet. Upon delivery to the sterile area, you note the item touches the outer edge of the wrap. Have the item removed, and the table area it contacted covered with a sterile towel. Again, debate is absurd.

3. Treat each patient as you would like to be cared for yourself. (Think about this for a moment: You would want the best work performance, and you would allow for no mistakes.) Practice this at all times.

Time is an important factor in operating room work. There is constant mention of time during the working day. But do not be overwhelmed by it. Those who keep "pushing" you still consider time secondary to approved aseptic technique. *For example:*

1. No one who tells you to set up as quickly as possible for an emergency operation wants you to sacrifice sterility. That person would sincerely want you to take the time necessary, if it meant a choice between a table that was sterile or unsterile, or an operating room that was complete or incomplete.

2. Picture this situation: During a surgical procedure, the drape near the operative field becomes damp. The nurse is occupied passing interrupted sutures to the surgeon, and the hands of both pass over the damp drape. In this case, the nurse's desire to please the surgeon has become stronger than her conscience toward technique. The surgeon depends on the nurse to recognize the contamination, and to take the time to remedy it. No surgeon wants a nurse to "keep up to his speed" on an unsterile field.

Professional honesty covers a wide scope. In an operating room, many errors other than breaks in aseptic technique occur. All these errors adversely affect the patient.

In the examples in Table 2-1, your lack of professional honesty perhaps lets you "get through another case." But it's you who causes the complications.

Table 2-1
EFFECTS OF LACK OF PROFESSIONAL HONESTY

Errors the nurse is aware of	*Lack of honesty*	*Result*
Mistake in solution	You hope the surgeon does not realize the solution is water instead of saline.	The skin graft may not "take" successfully.
Passing 3-0 silk instead of 2-0 silk	You pray the 3-0 silk will not break when tied.	The hernia recurs.
Losing a needle	The surgeon may never know since you reported the count as correct.	A perforated viscus makes a second operation necessary.

The nurse who passes instruments to the surgeon plays a vital part in successful surgery. Your honesty is paramount. Fear of reprimand is misplaced and insignificant compared with the catastrophic results to which your mistakes can lead. Have character enough to face your shortcomings.

INTEREST IN WORK

You must acquire interest in your work. That's the only way you will increase your knowledge of surgery. *For example:*

1. When assigned to an operation that is new or vague to you, seek information *before* the time of surgery. To be of value during a procedure, you must know the anatomy involved and the method of surgery employed. In order to gain the information, you can do the following:
   a. Refer to books.
   b. Have a team conference.
   c. Ask your supervisor to hold an in-service session.
   d. Jot down notes—this gives you reference material for the future.

2. When the operation is performed, the surgeon can sense your interest, and this will prompt him to show you anatomical structures and explain the procedure. On the other hand, if he senses your lack of interest, he will feel there is nothing to be gained by teaching you.

3. Your complete and constant interest in mastering details, even the smallest, is reflected in your speed and efficiency in more complex surgery. Do not form poor habits, such as:

a. Neglecting communication to a fellow team member.
b. Setting up the tables in a slipshod manner.
c. Taking shortcuts and not conforming to standard setups.
d. Preparing too much suture ahead of time (creates waste, and does not increase your speed).
e. Placing several instruments for the surgeon to choose from on the operative field (you should anticipate which one he will want next).
f. Forgetting to check the instrument basket for completeness and correct order.

Keep your standards high at all times. Do not allow yourself to reach a point where you are bored or above doing the small or common surgical procedures. Let any situation become a challenge to your skill, speed, and optimum delivery of patient care. *For example:*

1. Scrubbing for an inguinal herniorrhaphy. Try to recognize the sac when the surgeon does. Realize at which point the defect is ready to be closed. Know the method of closure, such as ligature, suture ligature, or pursestring. Know the type of repair the surgeon favors. Pass sutures of the correct length and strength at the proper time without his having to ask for them.

2. Circulating for a lipoma excision under local anesthesia. Realize the patient's anxiety, and put the patient at ease with communication and touch contact. Preserve the patient's privacy. Explain what you are doing, e.g., when moving him to the OR bed, monitoring vital signs, etc. Confirm that the

surgeon's requests have been addressed, and assure that the scrub assistant has the proper supplies—so you are free to comfort the patient.

If you can anticipate the surgeon's needs and have employed your utmost skill and speed; if you have decreased the trauma and anxiety of a patient's surgical experience; then you have met the challenge. How can you feel that the frequent surgical procedure is routine? Every case varies in some manner. There is always something to keep you interested, if only you would look for it.

ECONOMICAL USE OF HOSPITAL EQUIPMENT

It is a nurse's professional responsibility to give the best service, with the best equipment, at the lowest of operating costs. That does not mean to economize at the expense of safety. Safety must never be lost in an attempt to save money.

Hospital supplies are costly items. Your attitude toward these investments can either save money or upset the operating room budget. It is part of your job to respect the equipment you are given to work with. Careless use of equipment costs money. To offset this loss, hospital rates must be raised, or the operating room budget has less purchasing power. Either alternative affects you and the patients. *For example:*

1. Investigate the cost of a surgical gut (catgut) tie reel, a vascular suture, or an ophthalmic suture. How many have you opened unnecessarily? Estimate the dollars lost throughout the OR during a given day.

2. Investigate the cost of surgical gloves. How many were discarded because size was not confirmed?

3. Investigate the replacement or repair cost of a damaged cystoscope. Would prior knowledge of its proper use and care have prevented such fiscal loss? Will the next patient's care and hospital stay be affected because of lack of such an instrument?

4. Take time to study the waste and expense that goes on every day. Then be constructive with your criticism, and suggest means of preventing such loss.

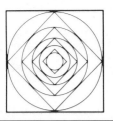

Chapter 3

Prevention of Infections

The prevention of infections is the responsibility of the entire surgical team. Prevention includes not only the use of aseptic techniques and careful sterilization of supplies, but also the practice and maintenance of aseptic conditions in the operating room. *Enforced* strict rules of conduct and dress, which apply to *all* persons using the facilities, and adequate disinfection of the room and used supplies are of paramount importance. A low infection rate is a credit to the professional staff, and also to the environmental services (porters) and auxiliary help. All are vital members of the preventative team. All must maintain the same standard of excellence in caring for each patient.

In considering the prevention of infections, there are two important points to bear in mind:

1. Our atmosphere contains bacteria, both pathogenic (disease-producing) and nonpathogenic.

2. When a prime barrier to infection—the skin—is broken, either by incision at the operation, or by trauma or an accident, the susceptibility to bacterial invasion is increased.

Bacteria do not "fly"; but when we realize that the harborers of bacteria, such as dust, and nose and throat droplets, are readily carried along by air currents (known as *airborne contamination*), we can visualize how easily a wound can be invaded. Take time to think of what actually happens when there is unnecessary activity in the room, or when a team member pulls off his mask while assisting in the transfer of a patient to the stretcher. Certainly the atmosphere of the OR environment is being affected.

The operating room staff must be vigilant in order to eliminate pathogens and keep the environmental bacterial count down. The following is a list of points of which all OR personnel should be aware. As you read each one, think about the reasons behind it.

1. No one who has a cold or infection is permitted in the operating room.

2. Personnel, doctors, ancillary help, and all people present in the OR suite must follow the rules regarding the special operating room dress code.

3. An adequate cap must be worn to cover the hair. Beards must also be covered (a special hood design is available).

4. Shoe covers are essential. Keeping one pair of shoes for OR use only is a chance situation, since the cleanliness of the shoes is questionable.

5. Operating room attire must be changed (or prop-

erly covered) before leaving the suite and on return. Head caps, masks, and shoe covers must be removed.

6. Masks are to be changed between operations. The choice of an efficient mask (properly worn) is important.

7. Conversations during surgery should be kept to a minimum.

8. Personnel must give proper attention to inadvertent cuts, needle pricks, eye splashes, etc.

9. Good scrub techniques must be employed. Attention to fingernails and skin crevices should be stressed. Use of good friction, proper detergent, and proper rinsing is essential. Scrub technique rules should be posted for all to follow.

10. When scrubbing, personnel should stay at the scrub sink area, as the procedure causes gross dissemination of bacteria. Logically, if you walk into a room during a procedure, you are contaminating the room, let alone not concentrating on the scrub technique.

11. Completion of sterilization of supplies should be ensured. (Observe sterilizer graph readings, color of pressure-sensitive tape, integrity of wrapping materials—no holes or tears, etc.—condition of chemical indicator in pack.)

12. The circulating nurse is required to wash her hands frequently.

13. When using a glove or sponge stick to handle contaminated supplies (e.g., picking up a used sponge

from the floor), the gloved hand should not be used to open a clean supply, nor the sponge stick placed by clean supplies.

14. All members must practice good aseptic technique. Recognize breaks and remedy them immediately.

15. The following aseptic techniques must be practiced in the sterile area:
    a. Exercise care at all times.
    b. Always face the sterile field to prevent accidental contamination.
    c. Never walk between two sterile fields.
    d. Do not set up cases for operation near a doorway (to avoid accidental contamination).
    e. Do not lean over, or reach arms over, the sterile field.
    f. When scrubbed, keep arms flexed at the elbow, and do not drop hands down.
    g. Protect gloved hands with a towel while awaiting the surgeon.

16. Personnel should always allow for a wide margin of safety.

17. The patient skin shave (removal of hair) should not be done in the room of surgery.

18. The antiseptic skin preparation of the patient must be adequate.

19. Clean cases should not follow infected cases, unless the room, equipment, etc., have been properly cleansed (decontaminated). The recommended practice is to treat all cases as if they were infected, thereby preventing cross-contamination from unknown sources.

20. Rooms, furniture, lights, and equipment must be cleaned after every case. Use the method prescribed by your hospital (e.g., germicide-detergent, wet vacuum).

21. Ventilating systems, room locations, and exchange areas should be studied, and the knowledge of them applied, wherever possible, to contribute to the prevention of infection.

22. Traffic into and out of the operating room must be kept to a minimum. Doors must be kept closed.

23. Unauthorized personnel are not allowed in the operating room.

24. Proper orientation of staff concerning rules should be provided, with the insistence that all persons abide by them.

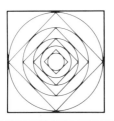

Chapter 4
Safety

Hospitals are constantly on the alert to provide safe conditions for the patients and for all who visit and work within their confines. Safety in the operating room encompasses not only the physical plant and the environment, but also the supplies, equipment, and techniques used for the surgical patient. Logically, the personnel must be knowledgeable of "safety practices" and "practice safety" at all times. Each chapter of this book promotes safe practices. This chapter highlights some important procedures that are part of the total safety plan.

PHYSICAL PLANT
EMERGENCY SITUATIONS

Procedures for physical plant emergency situations may vary from one hospital to another. Therefore, you must be familiar with the specific safety plan that is followed in your hospital, as well as the location of pertinent safety equipment.

Fire and disaster. Each institution has planned what to do in case of a fire or disaster. The fire and disaster manuals contain the procedural plan for each department, thereby preventing confusion in the event of one of these occurrences. Each *department* is responsible for posting the manuals in a visible area. Each *employee* is responsible for knowing the plans.

Knowing where the manuals are—but not having read them—courts danger. Not knowing the OR activities in effect at the time of such incidents is unforgiveable. To be prepared in the event of a fire:

1. Review the general hospital procedure, so you can be of help in the OR or in any area to which you may be dispatched for assistance.

2. Discuss with your supervisor the procedures pertinent to the OR. *For example:*
   a. If the fire is in the kitchen (even though it is several floors away), do not call for the next patient.
   b. Survey the number of patients present and the stage of each patient's operative procedure, and make sure that the OR teams are aware of the hospital alert.

3. Know where the alarm boxes are located in the OR (generally next to an exit).

4. Know the location of water hoses and fire extinguishers. Know what type extinguisher is available (e.g., electrical, paper).

5. Do not use elevators or transport patients from the OR or recovery room to the nursing units until the "all clear" is sounded.

6. Close doors. (Now do you realize why "propping" certain fire doors open is against the rules?)

   Disaster can be many things. It can be internal or external. The latter brings many patients requiring surgery to the hospital. To be prepared in the event of a disaster:

1. Know the internal disaster procedure and the routes for evacuation of patients.

2. Know the external disaster procedure (e.g., elective surgery is usually canceled, control officers need reports to know how many teams are available, personnel may be called in).

Bomb threat.   Today, hospitals have a procedure to follow in the event of a bomb threat. Read the procedure, and respond to the instructions (e.g., assist with search, evacuate patients).

Power outage.   Most ORs are on emergency power, and hospitals periodically test the system. To be prepared in the event of a power outage:

1. Inquire as to what equipment and electrical outlets are and are not on emergency power.

2. Know the location of flashlights. Check their working ability daily.

Water-leakage flood.   Unfortunately, all buildings are prone to such occurrences. Pipes do break, and a blockage in the sewage system does cause flooding. If the OR is located under a nursing unit, malfunctions in the

latter's plumbing and sewage systems can cause overhead leaks. In the event of water leakage or flood:

1. Check for the source.

2. Alert the proper department (e.g., maintenance).

3. Move equipment away from the leak (or use protec-
   tive covers). Lift equipment from the floors.

4. Avoid electrical contact.

Pressure (gas, oxygen, vacuum) alarms.   Modern ORs
with piped in gases, etc., have alarm boxes that contain pressure gauges, and are equipped to sound an
alarm and light a red light when the pressure falls
below safe readings. In the event the alarm goes off,
check to see which gas or vacuum is affected. Then:

1. Immediately notify maintenance.

2. Immediately notify the anesthesiologist and room
   teams of pressure inadequacy—they can resort to
   use of the adjunct tanks on the machines.

3. If vacuum (suction) is the problem, bring portable
   suction to the rooms, and summon extras from central service.

4. When the pressure problem is solved, report back to
   the anesthesiologist and room teams.

Hazard alarm.   Modern ORs are equipped with an
electrical device that detects a short circuit. When a
piece of electrical equipment has a short circuit, the
alarm emits a "buzzing" sound and activates a small
red light. A short circuit spells *danger*, and the following steps should be taken:

1. Immediately investigate the cause of the alarm activation.

2. Stop using the culprit equipment. Replace it with a substitute.

3. Alert the supervisor or control desk nurse.

4. Request immediate evaluation (or repair) by the biomedical department, maintenance, or the manufacturer of the equipment.

OTHER SAFETY CONSIDERATIONS

In addition to preparing for the above physical plant emergency situations, the following safety considerations should also be taken into account:

Waste anesthetic gas. There have been reports concerning the effects of trace anesthetic gases on the health of doctors and OR personnel. Consequently, the testing of room air, leak testing of anesthesia machines, and testing of amounts of gases at breathing zones should be routine safety activities. In addition:

1. Scavenging equipment is now used in the OR to suction out waste gases.

2. Preventive maintenance of anesthesia machines and equipment is an ongoing process.

X-ray. Radiologic procedures in the OR are commonplace. New equipment offers improved safety features in that the dispersing and bouncing of rays have been controlled. Nevertheless, it is still necessary that pre-

SAFETY PRACTICES

**The following is a short self-quiz concerning
everyday safety practices.**

Observe the scrub-up area:

1. Have you or someone else carelessly dripped soap and water on the floor, potentiating a slippery floor and consequent fall?

2. Do you request a mop-up when noticing a wet floor?

Observe the surgical room:

1. Is the furniture and equipment clean? Is it free from sharp, injurious points?

2. Do you check the suctions for proper functioning before each case?

3. Is there an orderly location of equipment? Can the patient stretcher enter without mishap? Are cabinet doors closed?

Think about electrical equipment. Do you:

1. Employ your basic knowledge of electricity?

2. Check cords for signs of fraying and exposed wires?

3. Avoid water contact? (For example: Just-sterilized "hot" electrical drills or devices must not be submerged in water for cooling purposes.)

4. Report defective electrical equipment?

5. Heed and act appropriately when the "hazard" alarm sounds?

Observe the access and egress areas:

1. Can a stretcher be moved easily, or is there clutter on both sides of the corridor?

2. Will hands be caught between the stretcher and doorway?

3. Will IV poles and auxiliary equipment strike overhangs, causing breakage of equipment and injury to patient or personnel?

cautions be taken by personnel for the safety of both personnel and the patient. *For example:*

1. Protection can be ensured by the use of lead aprons and lead shields (which you can stand behind).

2. Notice should be given to all persons (or a sign placed on the door indicating equipment is in use), so that unprotected people will not enter the room.

3. X-ray exposure can be monitored by what is referred to as an "X-ray badge." Persons, particularly those subjected to long-term X-ray or fluoroscopy procedures, should wear the badges. X-ray badges are individually assigned and worn by the particular person. They are collected monthly and tested or observed for degree of exposure readings. Any abnormal readings (above safe limits) are investigated.

4. Available gonad shields should be placed on patients, when appropriate.

Sterilizer (steam). The precautions applied to steam sterilization are as follows:

1. Proper biological monitoring must be done on a regimented schedule (see Chapter 5).

2. Burns can be avoided by knowing that:
   a. Metal doors absorb heat and are extremely hot after a sterilizing cycle.
   b. A residual amount of steam remains in the chamber at cycle completion. When opening the door, stand to the side—*not in front*—of the chamber.

3. Sterilization will not be achieved if:
   a. Pressure (pounds) and temperature (degrees) do not reach prescribed levels.

b. Items are not clean, instrument ratchets are not open, articles are improperly placed, or the sterilizer is overloaded.

Sterilizer (ethylene oxide gas). When sterilizing with a gas agent, read directions for operation and the precautions to be taken. *For example:*

1. Sterilizers must have an adequate venting cycle. Always wait for full cycle completion before opening the door.

2. Supplies must then be transferred to an aerator, hands protected in the process.

3. Manufacturers differ in time specifics, etc.

4. Biological monitoring is essential.

5. Remember that the plastic-type material used for packaging, the chemical indicators, and the pressure-sensitive tape differ from that used for steam sterilization.

Note: Certain materials other than metal (e.g., tubing) absorb gas. Consequently, if the patient was in contact with a gas-absorbed article (that had not been properly aerated), his life would be endangered.

SUMMARY

The operating room must be "safe" for the patients, physicians, nurses, and other personnel. Regulations must be established, clearly outlined, understood, and followed. It is essential that they be monitored by everyone.

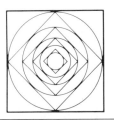

Chapter 5
Equipment

The term "equipment" refers to all items used in an operating room. Hospitals provide the surgical staff with as much equipment as their resources will allow. The value of the equipment, in money, is high, but the value to the patient and the staff must be measured by a different scale. A piece of equipment, if given proper care, if its qualities and purpose are understood, and if it is used correctly, increases in worth. In contrast, a piece of equipment is superfluous when it is mal-treated, and its purpose and use are vague to the staff.

It is essential that you know the equipment the institution has supplied the staff to work with. Sound and fast execution of the procedures depends upon the staff's knowledge of the location and use of the articles. You cannot always rely on others to be around to tell you where seldom-used items are located or whether, in fact, they are available. Nor can you wait until you are called upon to use a piece of equipment, to learn how it is correctly operated.

During the period of your orientation to an operating room, you will be taken on a tour. This will give you a general idea of the extent of available equipment. Use your own initiative, when slack moments are present, to investigate cupboards, inventories, and instructions for use. As new items are purchased, know where they are located, how to use them, how they are sterilized or made ready for use, and how they are cleaned and stored.

When you go to another hospital, you will not always find the same items you are accustomed to using. Find out in which way the equipment you know is supplemented by other items, and get acquainted with them. By doing that, you become a valuable member of a staff.

The fast pace of research and specialization provides the surgeon with a variety of materials for treatment. The existence of prosthetic appliances of all sizes and purposes illustrates the importance of knowing the physical properties of the product and of following the manufacturer's instructions. *For example:*

1. Orthopedic femoral head prostheses or fixation devices must be protected from scratches. Body fluids may react on the surface, causing corrosion and subsequent failure of the device.

2. Certain medical-grade silicone implant materials must be carefully handled, using gloves at all times, and protected from any lint. (Lint can cause foreign-body reactions.) Read and follow the manufacturer's directions.

3. Eye lens (intraocular) implants must be handled and treated with extreme care, and never touched— except by the surgeon, using forceps (under a mi-

croscope). The lens is irrigated with BSS (balanced salt solution) to remove any static.

DISPOSABLE EQUIPMENT

Today, many OR items are being replaced by similar, disposable products. They are evaluated by your supervisor on an individual basis. Consider the following with regard to disposable products:

1. They may be a good substitute—or a poor one, due to poor packaging or limited performance.

2. The cost may be prohibitive.

3. They are an economy to hospitals because they are laborsaving, but they are an expense to hospitals when carelessly handled, overstocked, and incompetently used.

4. They are a time-saver in operating rooms because of convenient packaging and sterility readiness, but cause time loss if proper opening of the packet is not understood or practiced.

Note: Disposable products are just what they state—disposable. This indicates that they are manufactured for *one* use and then discarded (disposed of). For example, a disposable cautery pencil is not made to withstand resterilizing; hence, it would be dangerous to use if it were resterilized.

REUSABLE EQUIPMENT

There are many kinds of reusable equipment found in the OR. Some are machines (e.g., anesthesia), some are motors (e.g., orthopedic drills), and some are permanently installed or are mobile (e.g., microscopes, X-ray apparatus, lead shields). Some reusable equipment requires disposable or reusable components (e.g., cautery). Be guided by the following:

1. Know how the equipment works, and learn the principles involved in its operation—including safety measures.

2. Know what component parts or accessories are necessary.

3. Assure that reusable and disposable components are available and ready for use—and report any decreases in inventory.

4. Assure the return of equipment to the proper storage area, and make certain that it is clean and ready for reuse.

5. Report any functional problems to your supervisor. Do not use equipment if there is obvious danger of malfunction.

ELECTROSURGICAL GENERATOR (CAUTERY)

The cautery, an electrosurgical generator, is a fre quently used piece of equipment. Therefore, it is worthy of explanation.

By means of a high-frequency electrical current, a cautery can cut, coagulate, and also cut and coagulate at the same time. It offers advantages for hemostasis, and can be used in areas where bleeding is difficult to control, e.g., endoscopic surgery (procedures done through a scope—transurethral prostatectomy, laparoscopy). The cautery can also reduce the dissemination of disease cells.

However, to be advantageous, the cautery must be in proper working order, its accessory parts must be inspected for flaws, and the operator(s), including the nurse who prepares it for use, must thoroughly understand the principles of electricity, as well as the safe operation of the machine. The principles of electricity, as applied to use of the cautery, are as follows:

1. The high-frequency electrical current comes from the cautery and passes through an active cable to the patient via a pencil-like instrument. The current passes through the patient and returns to the electrosurgical unit by means of a dispersive electrode (grounding pad) and cable.

2. Electricity cannot flow without a complete circuit.

3. If the grounding pad (dispersive electrode)—which is used with the cautery to make a complete circuit— is not properly placed on the patient, and if, for example, a metal table part such as a leg holder is not padded (insulated), the electricity may exit flow to that part and create a burn.

4. If the insulation on an endoscopic instrument is cracked, burns or shocks to the patient can result.

You can begin to see the vigilance required to operate an electrosurgical unit. It is your responsibility to know the many factors of safe cautery use. Logically, you must review them with your supervisor, and take time to read literature about the machine and the accessories. Be aware, it is not uncommon to use accessories from different manufacturers. Explanation in the use of the cautery is lengthy, and the following list gives you only some of the basic considerations for thought:

1. Machines and accessories must be approved and periodically checked by the biomedical department.

2. Always inspect instrumentation (endoscopes, pencils, etc.) before use.

3. Place the grounding pad on the patient *after* the patient has been placed in operative position.
   a. Avoid bony prominences, scar tissue, and areas with an inordinate amount of hair.
   b. Place the pad reasonably close to the preposed operative surgical site.
   c. Be sure the grounding pad is protected from liquids such as prep solution.
   d. Confirm good adherence. "Tenting" (section lifted up) can cause a request for higher power (because of poor grounding), and a severe burn can result.
   e. Check the site periodically; also check the condition of the patient's skin when the pad is removed post-surgery.
   f. Set the power controls at the proper levels (the usually adequate settings will have previously been determined).
   g. Be sure accessories are firmly attached to the machine.
   h. Protect the patient from undesired return paths of electricity (e.g., insulate metal table parts, assure that ECG electrodes are not near the area where the active "pencil" electrode will be used).

i. If the cautery is not working, check all accessories for proper connection and placement. Request your supervisor's inspection or assistance. You may need to change to a new machine.

STERILIZERS

It is imperative that you learn the proper use of sterilizers. Hospitals vary in their choice of manufacturer; hence, there is a variation of style. The basic principles are the same, but the mode of operation (e.g., buttons to be pushed, handles to be turned) differs. Your responsibility is to study the manuals, know the principles, and learn how to operate the equipment. Give attention to the dial readings—know how to interpret the readings and how to interpret the graph recordings—and be aware of the necessary time-temperature requirements for the article(s) to be sterilized.

Testing the efficiency of the sterilizer is done on a routine basis, and the test reports must be kept on file.

Three types of sterilizers, and the methods used to test them, are as follows:

1. Gravity-displacement steam sterilizers—usually found within the suite and commonly referred to as "flash" sterilizers (although the word "flash" is a misnomer)—must be spore tested at least once a week. This is referred to as "biological monitoring."

   Explanation: Non-spore-forming bacteria are more easily killed, and using such organisms for a test would not be a sufficient "challenge" for the sterilizer. Spore-forming bacteria are more difficult to kill, the *Bacillus stearothermophilus* being the most difficult to kill by steam. This particular spore is used to test steam sterilizers. Special inoculated spore strips or plastic ampules of inoculated media (e.g., Attest) are used (according to directions), and are sent to the specific laboratory or designated areas equipped for test evaluation.

2. Pre-vacuumed steam sterilizers use the same test. However, if the sterilizers are used for sterilizing wrapped supplies on a daily basis, they are tested more often. Pre-vacuumed sterilizers are also tested daily to confirm proper function, using a Bowie Dick test (this is not a spore test).

3. Gas (ethylene oxide) sterilizers undergo spore testing (usually on an each-load basis). However, the *Bacillus subtilis* is the bacterium of choice for gas sterilizers. *B. stearothermophilus* is easily killed by gas and, therefore, would not offer a "challenge."

Additional factors concerning the use of sterilizers are as follows:

1. Gas-sterilized supplies must undergo an adequate aeration process before they can be safely used in surgery.

2. The pressure-sensitive tape used to fasten packs turns color to indicate *sterilizing conditions* were met. It is important to know that the tape does not monitor the time-temperature exposure. The tape used to fasten packs for steam sterilization differs from that used for gas sterilization.

3. The chemical indicator located inside packs to indicate that the steam or gas has penetrated that area also differs in accordance with whether the sterilizer is gas or steam.

EMERGENCY EQUIPMENT

Time is of the essence when there is a patient crisis. ORs have equipment accessible and available—ready to go. The problem is having the personnel knowledgeable of the resuscitation procedures.

A patient crisis can occur in the waiting area, in surgery, or during transport to the recovery room. Emergency equipment includes:

1. *Ambu bag*—a means of respiratory resuscitation. It is available in adult as well as pediatric and infant sizes. The location should be known by the staff— usually prominently displayed or located with or on the "crash cart." Take time to:
   a. Read instructions for use.
   b. Practice attaching the face mask to the bag.
   c. Assure that the equipment is clean, complete, and actually present at its known location.

2. *Crash cart*—a cart that contains the equipment and drugs necessary for cardiac resuscitation. In addition, it may contain instrument sets—or gear—for other emergencies, such as emergent tracheostomy. It often has particular charting records that facilitate the recording of information during an emergent (code) situation. The locations of its inner contents are arranged to *save time*. Being so equipped, it can be readily moved to the requested location so that the needed supplies are at your fingertips. Learn the contents of the crash cart and when and how they are used. Contents include:
   a. Defibrillator with external paddles. (Sterile internal paddles are also available.)
   b. Drugs arranged in labeled sections.

c. Needles and syringes, IV solutions and tubing, dressings and tape.

d. Items for respiratory problems (laryngoscope, endotracheal tubes of various sizes, etc.).

You have a responsibility to:

- Know the cart contents.
- Know how to use the defibrillator.
- Keep accurate records of the time of code, drug name, dosage, time of administration, and outcome of code.
- Restock the cart and assure cleanliness.
- Check expiration dates of drugs and sterility expiration date of instrument trays.
- Check the working order of the defibrillator—daily.

CASE CARTS

Case carts are new pieces of equipment that are now found in many ORs. They are part of a system designed to facilitate the procurement of basic supplies needed for a case, decrease downtime between cases, and release the professional nurses from nonprofessional duties. By formulation of basic requisitions for cases, central service or OR aides can gather the supplies and stock the carts. The nurse no longer has to go back and forth for setup packs, drapes, sponges, etc. Consider the following information concerning the case cart system:

1. It does not eliminate the need for procuring suture and special supplies for the individual case and patient needs.

2. It does create an orderly preparation for a case.

3. Used supplies go back on the cart for disposition in the soiled workroom or central service.

4. Unused supplies are delivered to the collection area.

5. The room itself is vacated post-surgery in a more orderly manner.

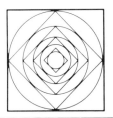

Chapter 6

Drugs and Solutions

Drugs and solutions are required for the basic cleaning of the operating room; for the preparation of the surgical setup; for the scrub procedure of the operative team; for the skin preparation of the patient; as medications used during the operation; and for cleaning the room and equipment after the operation. Hospitals and physicians vary in their choice of drugs and solutions. Nevertheless, basic needs must be met, in relation to both the performance and quality of the drugs and solutions involved.

In the operating room you are constantly entrusted with the use of drugs and solutions. For the patient's safety—and your own—and in order to be an intelligent and trustworthy surgical team assistant, you must understand and consider the factors affecting the use of drugs and solutions. The following points will serve as a guide.

DISINFECTING SOLUTIONS

Know the names and qualities of solutions used to disinfect by chemical means. *For example:*

1. Select the solution according to the item that is being disinfected.
   a. Some solutions dissolve finishes and enhance rust.
   b. Some solutions cause corrosion.
   c. Some materials absorb the disinfecting chemical (e.g., certain plastics, conductive rubber anesthesia masks), and tissue injury or skin irritation will occur on contact with the material.
   d. Solutions vary in their effectiveness against different bacteria.

2. Know the percentage strength of the solution.
   a. A solution that is overdiluted will not achieve disinfection.
   b. To use a stronger solution than necessary is wasteful (or possibly ineffective, as in the case of alcohol).

3. Know the time necessary to achieve disinfection.
   a. Time varies with the solution employed and type of bacteria present.
   b. Prolonged soaking dulls sharp instruments.

4. Observe the expiration date of the solution.

5. Be aware that certain solutions (e.g., Cidex, Sporicidin) are activated by being mixed with an accompanying drug and that the effectiveness for disinfection is limited.
   a. At the time of activation, label the bottle with the expiration date. (Check literature for time.)

b. At the time of filling the solution boat, label the boat with the date that appears on the original bottle.

6. Know the terminology used in classifying disinfectants, as follows:
   a. *Bactericide*—agent capable of destroying bacteria. (Note: This does not mean *all* bacteria. It is imperative to know which specific bacteria a bactericide is effective against.)
   b. *Bacteriostat*—agent that inhibits the growth of bacteria. (Many of the surgical scrub soaps are bacteriostats.)
   c. *Sporicide*—agent capable of destroying spore-forming bacteria.

   Consider the following factors in using disinfecting solutions:

1. The article to be disinfected must be clean and free from any debris.

2. Complete submersion of the article is necessary. All surfaces of the article must be in contact with the solution.
   a. Instruments must be opened.
   b. If an instrument has several parts (e.g., cystoscope), they must be separated.

3. The receptacle must not be moved during the disinfecting process. Solution spilling up onto the sides of the receptacle causes contamination by washing bacteria back into the chemical agent. If this occurs, the time cycle must begin anew. (It is recommended that sterile receptacles be used, thereby increasing the margin of safety.)

4. Discretion must be applied when reusing solutions. (Observe the expiration date on the label, the condition of the solution, etc.)

5. The disinfecting solution must be thoroughly rinsed from all surfaces of the article before use. Use a sterile receptacle (boat) containing sterile distilled water.

6. Soaking ampules for disinfection is considered a dangerous process. An unrecognized crack in glass may allow the entrance of solution into medication, with resulting injury to the patient.

SKIN PREPARATION SOLUTION

Each institution has a routine procedure to render the operative site surgically clean. Procedure and choice of solution vary with the type of surgery and age of the patient. *For example:*

1. *Industrial accident.* Routine skin preparation is preceded by removal of gross dirt or irrigation of the wound.

2. *Cranial surgery.* The removal of hair is usually not done on the nursing unit, but in the operating room area. There is a special setup for removal of hair prior to entering the actual operating room. The condition of the scalp is a factor in the choice of skin preparation solution.

3. *Pediatric surgery.* The patient's sensitive skin may indicate the need for a special solution. Similarly, patients with *allergies* may require a change from routine preparation.

4. *Orthopedic surgery.* Routine procedure is revised to provide for additional skin preparation before coming to surgery, as well as in the operating room.

The following hazards are to be avoided:

1. Burns from strong solutions. Check the percentage strength of the solution you are using.

2. Injury to ears, eyes, and mucous membrane. These parts may have to be protected by cotton, towels, petrolatum, or gauze fluffs.

3. "Pooling" of solution. Solutions running down the arms or sides of the patient may accumulate and cause burns or skin irritation.

4. Use of improper solution. Use only the solution specified for the procedure. If an incorrect solution has been poured and used, report it immediately to the doctor, so that steps may be taken to rectify the error.

EMERGENCY DRUGS

When emergency situations occur in the OR, a successful patient outcome is dependent upon the prompt, knowledgeable action of the staff. That includes assuring the presence and orderly storage of the specific drugs needed for various patient emergencies. (Note: Drugs are only a part of the emergency treatment required; special equipment such as defibrillators, cooling blankets, iced intravenous normal saline, etc., is also essential in the treatment of life-threatening situations.) In the event of a patient emergency, the OR nurse is expected to:

1. Know the location of the supply of emergency drugs.

2. Know how a drug is administered, and bring the corresponding equipment (e.g., syringe) with the drug to the site.

3. Restock the emergency drugs and supplies after the emergency—even if it means staying overtime!

Note: At the time of an emergency, you cannot afford to lose a second. Therefore, it is logical that you accept responsibility for obtaining knowledge and completing tasks. Visualize what a detriment it would be if you did not know what the crash cart contained, or the location of the other emergency drugs, or, even worse, if you found that the emergency supply on the cart had not been restocked.

Examples of emergency situations are:

1. *Cardiac arrest.* This emergency, like all others, requires a team effort. The OR nurse must know the pertinent drugs used, and must develop dexterity in preparing them for the doctor.

2. *Malignant hyperthermia.* This is a medical emergency that may be precipitated by the use of anesthesia. Without prompt and appropriate treatment, the mortality rate may be as high as 70%.

3. *Anaphylaxis.* The drugs used for chemonucleolysis can produce an acute anaphylactic reaction.

Each of the above conditions requires prompt treatment. Consequently, ORs prepare for such emergency situations by having:

1. A crash cart containing the drugs necessary for the treatment of cardiac arrest.

2. Specific drugs available for treating malignant hyperthermia and for anaphylactic reaction to the drugs injected during chemonucleolysis. (Note: The drugs, necessary admixtures, and proper syringes and needles should be placed in individual boxes or kits and properly labeled, e.g., "malignant hyperthermia"; "chemonucleolysis reaction."

3. In-service sessions covering not only the drugs used, but also other specific requirements for treatment. Such sessions are vital in ensuring a thorough understanding of these untoward patient conditions.

DRUGS FOR
SPECIFIC SURGICAL PROCEDURES

Know which drugs are required for the procedure. *For example:*

1. Specific drugs are needed to accomplish local anesthesia (for eye, throat, and nerve surgery, etc.).

2. Specific drugs are employed in roentgen photography (cystogram, cholangiogram, etc.).

3. Specific drugs are used to prevent clotting of blood.

4. Specific antibiotic drugs may be indicated.

5. Specific drugs are used to aid hemostasis.

   Read procedural and doctor preference cards.

1. Obtain the required drugs and solutions at the time of preparation for the case (e.g., glycine for transurethral prostatic resection, balanced salt solution for ophthalmic procedure).

2. Know what vehicle is used for administration (e.g., TUR tubing set, syringe or irrigation tubing).

Have the drugs available for the procedure. Ask yourself:

1. Is the drug administered at sterile field? If so, prepare it, and have it ready for use by the surgeon.

2. Is the drug administered by the circulating nurse? If so, prepare it, and have it ready for use.

Note: In either case, do not discard the ampule or bottle. Keep it to show the label to the doctor before he uses the drug. That provides protection for the patient, the surgeon, and you.

Exercise care in the handling of drugs for roentgen photography (e.g., cholangiogram) at the operative field. Be sure the adapter fits securely on the syringe; otherwise:

1. Spillage will distort the X-ray, and the outline of the duct or organ will not be clearly defined.

2. The solution may be irritating to other tissues.

BASIC CONSIDERATIONS

Read the label three times. (Suggested procedure: Read the label as you are taking the drug or solution from the shelf or box; read it before you pour or draw the solution or drug into the syringe; and read it when you are replacing the drug on the shelf.)

1. Observe dosage strength.

2. Observe the expiration date.

3. Follow directions for use.

Keep drugs in order:

1. For easy selection.

2. To aid in daily ordering.

3. To prevent depletion of supply.

Note: Drugs for internal and external use should be stored separately.

Report low inventory levels.

1. Inform the charge nurse when you are using the last supply.

2. Suggest, if appropriate, a change in the par level.

Confirm the reasonable order of refrigerated drugs. Also, assure that the refrigerator temperature is between 36° and 46°F.

Learn the categories of drugs (e.g., anesthesia, ophthalmic, emergency), including:

1. Those drugs that must be refrigerated.

2. Narcotics and those controlled drugs for which special storage and accounting are required.

Be aware that your knowledge of drug supply, location, and expiration dates can be enhanced by your assisting in:

1. Cleaning the drug cabinets.

2. Ordering the drugs.

3. Checking in the pharmacy delivery.

Know the deterioration factor of drugs and solutions. Recognize changes due to:

- time
- heat
- cold
- light
- air
- moisture

Label syringes, cups, or medicine glasses containing drugs and solutions that are made ready prior to use. *For example:*

1. Suppose you have added the prescribed amount of heparin to 200 ml of sterile normal saline, for use in irrigation of the vessel in an embolectomy procedure. Label the bottle accordingly. If you leave the room and another nurse takes over your duties, there will be no question in her mind as to what is in the bottle.

2. Visualize yourself. You are scrubbed at the operative field and you know you will need, ready for use, a syringe of lidocaine and a syringe of heparin. Attach pre-sterilized labels to syringes, so there can be no error or last-minute confusion. (Labels can also be made by use of a sterile marking pen on Steri-strips, or the circulating nurse can use pencil on pressure-sensitive tape. Make a label and then sterilize it.)

Place medicine cups containing drugs in an emesis basin as a precaution in case they are inadvertently toppled, causing them to:

1. Spill on the table (potential contamination).

2. Spill into the open wound.

Have antidotes on hand for untoward effects of drugs, as can occur during the chemonucleolysis procedure, or due to allergic reactions to lidocaine or iodopyracet (Diodrast).

Keep informed about new drugs.

1. Read the brochure describing the drug.

2. Know its method of use in your institution.

3. If a new drug is used, report it to your supervisor, so that she can plan a teaching conference for the rest of the staff.

Chart medications used during surgery:

1. To inform the nurse on the patient care unit.

2. To assure that use of the medication is charged to the patient.

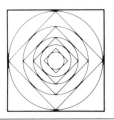

Chapter 7
Linen

Even though disposable nonwoven setup packs and drapes are available and popularly used because of certain superior qualities, linen is present in ORs in varying degrees. Some use it entirely for setup packs and draping; others use it to wrap instrument sets or selected items; almost all use huck towels. It is important for you to know the general care procedure for linen, and to understand the principles involved in the sterilization of packs—whether for setup packs or instrument sets.

BASIC CONSIDERATIONS

When folding linen for sterilization and, again, when using linen at the operative field, inspect for holes. In doing so:

1. You prevent contamination. (A hole in a sterile piece of linen defeats sterility of the field or enclosed article.)

2. You prevent "beyond-repair" damage of linen. (A small hole is mended more easily than a large tear.)

Note: The laundry or central service uses a light table to detect holes before linen is distributed for packs, drapes, or wrappers. Be aware that patches can fall off, and too many patches would indicate that the material is getting to the point of being "unfit for use."

A linen wrapper should be of double thickness, and the item double wrapped, to ensure safety. The circulating nurse, using proper aseptic technique, should open both wrappers. (Logically, the second wrapper is used in the event there is an undetected minute hole in the first wrapper. You would not want the scrub assistant, then, to touch the inner wrapper, decreasing the margin of safety.)

To assure sterility of linen packs, refer to regulations on sterilizer temperature and time, limitation of pack size, placement of contents in the pack, and position in the sterilizer. *For example:*

1. Sterilizing steam must penetrate the entire pack. Too large a pack, or one with heavy, solid items in the center, will deter this process.

Note: Placement of the "sterilizing *condition*" chemical indicator in the center of each pack is an added safety measure. It means that steam has penetrated the center, but the actual temperature and time of exposure, which would assure sterilization, are vague. Sterilizer efficiency can only be assured through regular periodic biological monitoring; sterility of supplies is assured through rigid regulations and constant observation of the graphic sterilizer charts by competent personnel.

2. Pans or basins in linen setup packs prevent the steam from penetrating the linen articles directly beneath.

3. Placement in the sterilizer and the time of exposure to sterilizing temperature vary according to the articles being treated and the type of sterilizer used (e.g., gravity-displacement or pre-vacuum steam sterilizers, or gas (ethylene oxide) sterilizer).

4. Packs must be dry before removal from a steam sterilizer. Wrapped items in a gas (ethylene oxide) sterilizer must be properly aerated.

After a designated length of time, the unused article is considered unsterile and unsafe (one month is the usual determined time for linen-wrapped supplies). Packs are labeled with the expiration date. *Remember*, misuse, improper storage, or dampness can render packs unsterile, regardless of any date on them. To ensure sterility of sterile linen held in storage:

1. Store sterile goods in a clean, dry area.

2. Rotate sterile supplies. (As sterile packs arrive for storage, place them in back of the present supply.) Use previously sterilized items first.

3. Avoid confusion. Never place "to-be-sterilized" bundles near sterile bundles.

4. Do not replace pressure-sensitive tape, or rewrap bundles that were opened unnecessarily (they must be sterilized again).

5. If a sterile pack is opened and not used, take it apart and send the linen items to the laundry—even though they are clean. Laundering replenishes mois-

ture to the fabric, bringing the fibers closer together. If not laundered, but sterilized repeatedly, linen turns brownish, and becomes porous and unsafe for use in surgery.

6. Store linen supplies away from solutions. That applies to storage in cabinets and to extra linen held ready during an operation. Sterile packs must be stored on shelves above those containing solutions (e.g., saline, antiseptics). Doing so:
   a. Prevents the possibility that supplies will become damp and, therefore, contaminated.
   b. Saves time and labor of co-workers, who have to resterilize the bundles you have carelessly handled.

Sterile supplies that fall to the floor must not be used, even though they are double wrapped. The desired margin of aseptic safety is jeopardized.

Shake out soiled linen before placing it in the laundry hamper, in order to:

1. Prevent loss of equipment.

2. Prevent cuts or other injuries to ancillary workers by knife blades, etc.

Place wet linen in the center of discarded dry linen, to prevent the linen hamper from getting wet, thus avoiding the consequent spread of contamination.

Lengthen the life of linen items. *For example:*

1. Do not use good towels for cleaning furniture.

2. Do not expose linen to unnecessarily high temperatures for long periods of time.

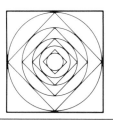

Chapter 8
Instruments

SELECTING INSTRUMENTS FOR AN
OPERATIVE PROCEDURE

There are different ways to select and assemble a basket of instruments for an operative case. One method you may choose to follow is to say to yourself: "Knife, scissors, forceps, clamps, retractors, and special needs." Another way is to visualize the operation step by step, and select the instruments in order of their use. The placement of instruments in the basket must conform to the pattern established in your particular operating room. The type and quantity of instruments depend on the case at hand. The following information will assist you in selecting the needed instruments.

PURPOSE OF INSTRUMENTS

Each instrument is designed to do a specific job. The many variations are necessary to cope with the location, size, depth, and function of the anatomical structure. For efficient results, an instrument must be employed for the purpose for which it has been fashioned. Examples of instruments used in operative procedures, along with their particular characteristics and functions, are listed below.

1. Knives (scalpels)
   a. The commonly used scalpel is actually a knife handle used with sharp, removable, disposable blades. The handle may be short or long, and the blade varies (rounded edge, slanted point, narrow shaft, etc.), to accommodate the location and type of tissue to be cut. For example, the blade needed to excise a nevus would be of delicate design, compared with the blade used for an abdominal incision on an adult.
   b. There are some surgical knives of one-piece construction. Extreme care in handling this permanent blade is imperative to preserve the sharpness and avoid nicks; it must be meticulously inspected before use.

   Examine scalpel handles and the various blades. Practice safely placing a blade on the handle, and then safely removing it.

2. Forceps
   a. *Plain thumb forceps* are non-traumatic in design. The tips may be blunt or tapered (the tissue involved determines your selection). The plain tips avert injury to underlying anatomical structures, as well as trauma to the grasped structures. (They are used to pick up peritoneum, intestine, blood vessels.)
   b. *Tooth tissue forceps* enable the surgeon to grasp tissue firmly and, at the same time, exert ten-

sion. The teeth vary in number and length (the tissue involved determines your selection). Tooth tissue forceps must be used with caution because of their traumatizing effect. (They are used on skin, scar tissue, muscle.)

3. Scissors
   a. *Heavy pattern scissors* are more efficient on resistant or dense tissue.
   b. *Fine scissors* are best employed on tissue requiring meticulous dissection.
   c. *Suture scissors* are designed to cut sutures. *Wire scissors* are designed to cut wire. Other scissors are ruined if employed for those purposes. Examine the various scissors and realize the proper care they deserve.

4. Clamps
   a. The varied designs meet specific purposes. They may be used for hemostasis or to grasp tissue for retraction.
   b. The same safety rule applies to clamps as to forceps: The clamp with a tooth (Kocher, Allen, Ochsner) must be used with caution.

Familiarize yourself with the selection of clamps available at your hospital and their possible usages. For example, many institutions refer to a certain clamp as a "gallbladder clamp." Actually, it may be a Lower gall duct forceps. The essential and significant factors are the angle and depth of the design. Knowing that, use your initiative, and have such clamps available for other cases where depth at an angle is involved, e.g., in the usual nephrectomy setup. The Lewis tonsil hemostat can supplement the Adson clamps on hand for chest surgery. Depth and angle are, again, the determining factors.

5. Retractors
   a. Retractors are *usually used in pairs* to provide even exposure by walling off surrounding tissue.
   b. A retractor can be a single instrument—*self-retaining*. The blades of the instrument open and stay in place to retract the tissue.
   c. Retractors *vary* in size, shape, and flexibility to meet a given situation.
   d. There are *special designs* for specific situations: A Burford Finochietto is designed to retract a rib cage; a Ragnell (double-ended) retractor allows a choice of small blade size for areas of short depth.

Instruments are manufactured in various lengths, widths, and configurations. *Selection* depends on:

1. *Size of the patient* (baby, adult, obesity).

2. *Depth* of the operative site.

3. *Doctor's preference*.

4. *Anatomy* involved.

Examine some instruments at random and visualize the areas in which they could be used.

NUMBER OF INSTRUMENTS

The factors that determine the *quantity* of instruments needed are:

1. Size of the patient (baby, adult, obesity).

2. Anatomy involved. *For example:*

  a. Will there be a large initial skin incision?
  b. Will the incision be small and the entire proce-
     dure superficial?
  c. Will the operation be in a very vascular area?
  d. Will the operation require a large variety of
     instruments?

3. Condition of the patient. *For example:*
  a. Accident case. Debridement followed by ortho-
     pedic surgery may require two separate setups
     of instruments.
  b. Septic case. Guard against taking a superfluous
     number of instruments into the operating room
     and subjecting them to contamination.

4. Special techniques. You need more instruments
   when the technique employed is to use an instrument *once* and pass it off for washing and resterili-
   zation (cancer technique).

5. Surgeon's preferences. *For example:*
  a. If a surgeon uses cautery for hemostasis, it may
     cut down on the number of instruments needed.
  b. A surgeon who uses clamps for retraction may
     require an extra supply.

INSTRUMENT SETS

Sets of instruments are assembled in baskets for particular operations, e.g., major, minor, intestinal, cata-
ract. Basic considerations regarding instrument sets
are that they:

1. Contain standard amounts of each type of instrument. Each instrument is counted (counts are discussed in Chapter 11).

2. Have standard arrangements.

The nurse is required to select the particular set(s) for the operative procedure; however, the surgeon's preference may require certain "extras." In such an instance:

1. Assure that the standard set is kept intact.

2. Handle the "extras" separately.

3. Do not encumber the standard set with "extras."

At the end of the procedure, the nurse should ensure that the set is complete and in the original order on return to the decontaminating room. Doing so:

1. Assures an accurate count.

2. Maintains proper supply of the set.

3. Decreases labor in the reprocessing area.

4. Confirms the nurse's regard for regulations and proper care of instruments.

PASSING INSTRUMENTS AT THE OPERATIVE FIELD

The following points are basic considerations in handling instruments. These points can be correlated with the teaching plan of any institution. Practice in your spare moments to attain speed and dexterity.

1. Use both hands. Time is saved by coordinating motion of both hands.
   a. The hand near the operative field passes most of the instruments to the surgeon. Have only one

kind of clamp in your hand at a time (this pre-vents loss of speed while switching to the desired clamp, and avoids confusion and unnecessary hazard).

  b. The hand near the sterile table is free to (1) re-ceive used instruments from the operative field, and to cleanse and replace instruments on the table; (2) resupply the stand above the operative field; and (3) pass a newly requested instrument not in the other hand.

2. Place instruments gently but firmly in the surgeon's hand. Keep your hand low and convenient to the operative field, so that:
  a. Your hand is on the same level as the surgeon's.
  b. Your motion is smoother.

3. *Do not dangle instruments near the surgeon's hand.*
  a. The surgeon does not want to take his eyes from the operative field to receive an instrument.
  b. Time is wasted when the passing of an instru-ment is not deliberate.

4. Although sterilized with ratchets opened, clamps should be closed on the first notch of the ratchet before passing them to the surgeon. Doing so:
  a. Keeps the instrument from becoming tangled with other instruments.
  b. Makes it easier for the surgeon to open the instrument.

5. Assist the surgeon's speed of operation when pass-ing an instrument. The handle must be free for placement in his hand, and the tip must be free for action.
  a. Pick up clamps and scissors at the joint, forceps

at the fused end, and retractors by the center portion, using your thumb and index finger. Thus, handle and tip are exposed.

b. Pick up a scalpel by the handle (just beyond the blade), with four fingers on one side, thumb on the other.

6. Protect the surgeon and yourself from injury due to sharp instruments.

a. When not in use, keep the scalpel on the instrument stand. If left on the field, it may fall to the floor (or on your foot), or the surgeon may reach for a sponge stick and accidentally grasp the cutting blade.

b. Never allow your hand to be beneath the scalpel blade, nor carelessly point the knife where the surgeon may accidentally strike the blade.

c. Exercise caution when handling instruments with hooks and prongs. They may "prick" a glove or penetrate a sterile drape.

7. Keep instruments clean.

a. A clamp is inefficient if there is tissue adhering to the tip.

b. A "bloody" clamp adheres to a surgeon's glove.

8. Change knife blades in a direction away from the field.

a. If you don't, your hand might slip, and the blade could fall into the wound or among instruments.

b. Doing so prevents unnecessary hazards to all concerned.

9. An instrument, knife blade, or needle that pricks or tears a glove must be discarded.

a. Change the glove—contaminated.

b. Discard the instrument, knife blade, or needle—
   contaminated.

PASS THE PROPER INSTRUMENTS
AT THE PROPER TIME

To be able to pass the proper instrument, you must keep your eyes on the operative field. That is the only way you can estimate the surgeon's needs. It enables you to keep up with unexpected changes or emergencies. Everyone knows it is the answer, but few have mastered the art. Nurses continually give more attention to the sterile table than to the operative field. The number of instruments, sutures, and supplies becomes overwhelming. Why? They are not always put in the same place, and the nurse keeps looking or rearranging to be sure where they are. That practice can be eliminated by routine setups.

Once habit patterns are established, the use of the complete setup becomes automatic. You can then reach toward the sterile table and pick up the desired article without taking your eyes from the operative field. In order to be able to pass the proper instruments at the proper time:

1. Learn the steps of the surgical procedure.

2. Have the proper instrument(s) ready at the proper time (anticipation).

3. Have the instrument ready for use. (Certain instruments have integrated parts that must be reassembled after sterilization.)

4. Be alert and, consequently, prevent instruments from falling to the floor.

CARE AND STORAGE OF INSTRUMENTS

To prolong their usefulness, surgical instruments should be properly stored and cared for. Remember the following:

1. Clean instruments thoroughly after use.
   a. Removal of tissue and excretions must be completed before sterilization.
   b. Instruments must be sterilized after use, and before storing, to protect staff.
   c. When instruments are not in use, all surfaces must be dry to prevent rust.

2. Sterilize instruments according to the institution's and manufacturer's recommendations.
   a. Instruments must be sterilized with ratchets opened. (Use of "pegs" in the instrument basket, or of specially designed bars or pins holds instruments open.)
   b. Each institution sets specific time limits (sterility expiration) and methods of sterilization. Follow regulations.
   c. The manufacturer advises when specific methods of care must be adhered to. Some instruments cannot withstand high steam temperatures (e.g., arthroscopes) and must be gas (ethylene oxide) sterilized. That promotes safety in care of the instrument.
   d. Certain sets (e.g., arthroscopy sets) require proper placement of articles in sterilizing cases to prevent damage to fib ·optic cords and delicate instrumentation.
   e. The safety practice of placing an indicator in the instrument basket can be an additional alert to a malfunctioning sterilizer.

3. Do not misuse or abuse instruments.
   a. All surgical instruments are precision instruments and must be treated accordingly. (For example, a Kelly clamp must not be used to tighten a faucet.)
   b. Prevent damage to dropped instruments by picking them up immediately; they are easily stepped upon and broken.
   c. Sharp or fine-edged instruments (e.g., osteotomes, iris scissors) are more delicate than other instruments, and require special attention. Store and sterilize them carefully.
   d. Instruments designed for ophthalmic or plastic surgery are taxed beyond their purpose if used in general surgery. The strain renders them useless in future special work.
   e. Careless stacking of instruments in the decontamination room is an obvious instrument abuse. A not-so-obvious example of misuse—that results in blatant abuse—is the practice of placing very bloody, tissue-laden instruments in a washer sterilizer. (The washing process may not remove all the sediment, and the heat of the sterilizing cycle can literally "cake" the debris onto the instruments.)

4. Prevent careless loss of instruments.
   a. Shake out drapes before placing them in the hamper.
   b. Remove clamps from specimens going to the laboratory, unless otherwise specified.
   c. Keep a record of instruments that were loaned to nursing units and of those that go back with surgical patients.

    d. Handle instruments having numerous parts carefully. When storing, check for completeness.

5. Repair instruments at the first sign of defect. The repair will cost less, and patients and doctors will not be subjected to imperfect instruments.

6. Return instruments to their proper place when not in use. It saves time for the staff and facilitates inventory. Also, it enables the new nurse to realize the extent of the instrument supply and the novice to learn the names of the instruments.

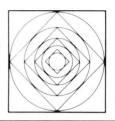

Chapter 9
Suture Material

Suture is defined as "the act, or operation, of uniting parts by stitching, as in surgery, or the thread or other material used in the operation."

Today, the uniting of parts is not limited to stitching, as with surgical thread. The surgeon now has other devices that have the ability to ligate vessels, or anastomose or close a wound. As a matter of fact, even small superficial wounds can be held closed by the use of sterile tape-like strips.

Selection of suture tends to confuse operating room nurses. Some confusion is decreased by use of the surgeon's preference card—but it is not the solution. A nurse's anxiety will be eased if she understands the purpose and accepted use of each type of suture material. It is a matter of knowing which suture material is qualified to meet the demands of the anatomy involved or the proposed procedure.

The wide range of regular suture material available today has not only given the surgeon an unlimited choice, but has allowed him to do advanced surgical procedures. For example, in microsurgery, there are sutures available that are finer than a strand of hair, and the swaged needle is minute in size. (Chapter 10 discusses suture needles.)

The physical characteristics of suture vary, not only in appearance, but in purpose, and even in required knotting techniques.

IDENTIFYING SUTURE MATERIAL

Companies vary in the processing and packaging of sutures. They label each suture with identifying company code numbers, and type (material) and size of suture. If a needle or needles are present, they provide a description (cutting, taper, etc.); list a needle identification number; and illustrate the needle(s). Some state an expiration date. Some even provide a dotted line to denote the direction to tear open the suture packet.

Sutures may be packaged "multi-strand" (more than one strand in the packet), or wound on reels (facilitates ligating superficial vessels—and is economical), or with swaged needles (needles attached to the suture). Sutures can be double armed (needle on each end), and more than one swaged suture may be included per packet. Some sutures have a "detach" (quick-release) needle.

An outer plastic cover of peel-away design protects the sterile suture packet. Suture packets come boxed with appropriate complete labeling, and are sometimes color coded.

It will add to your education and your performance, if you take time to examine the boxes and packets, and note the information on the labels. Some labels will state "general closure," "ophthalmic," "gastrointestinal," etc., which assists in correlating type and use of sutures. For example, you will note that ophthalmic sutures have cutting needles, while gastrointestinal sutures have taper needles.

Because of the large variety of available sutures (one type may be supplied with various sizes and kinds of needles), each suture is given a special code number. It is becoming increasingly necessary to learn code numbers, in order to facilitate quick selection from the shelf or rack.

CLASSIFICATION OF SUTURE MATERIAL

Suture material can be classified as follows:

1. Absorbable and nonabsorbable.

2. Natural and synthetic.

A natural, absorbable suture is surgical gut; a natural, nonabsorbable material is silk. Some synthetic materials are absorbable—Vicryl, Dexon, and PDS (polydioxanone); others are not—Prolene, nylon.

SIZE AND TENSILE STRENGTH
OF SUTURE MATERIAL

All sizes and tensile strengths are standardized by suture manufacturing companies according to specific regulations or standards.

Size denotes the diameter of the material. A system of numbers is used to identify it. *For example:*

1. The more zeros (0s) in the number, the finer the strand. But rather than labeling the packet 000000

(6 zeros), the accepted term is 6-0. This is a very fine suture.

2. As the number of 0s decreases, the size of the strand becomes larger. You arrive at 0, and then continue up 1, 2. There is a wide range of sizes. The trend is to use finer strands; #2 is not used often.

Tensile strength denotes the amount of pull that may be exerted on the strand before it breaks. Each size mentioned heretofore has a particular tensile strength. The finer the suture, the less tensile strength. For example, size 6-0 suture will break with less pull than that required to break size 0. Different materials have, of course, different tensile strengths (chromic 0 strength is different from 0 silk).

AVAILABLE SUTURE MATERIAL

Operating rooms attempt to standardize the sutures kept in stock. The many varieties and sizes of sutures make this economy imperative. When a suture that is not stocked in the OR is requested, report the request to your supervisor. There may be a similar suture available that can be substituted. If, however, the requested suture becomes actively used, it will be ordered. An outmoded type will probably be discontinued at the same time to prevent hospital funds from being tied up. You should:

1. Know the suture material stocked by the OR. No time will then be lost during the procedure by requesting a non-stocked item.

2. Report to the supervisor a surgeon's request for suture material not stocked by the hospital.

COMMONLY USED SUTURE MATERIAL

The "commonly" used sutures may vary from one hospital to another, depending on the surgical specialties—and, of course, the physician's choice. The names of the synthetic materials will vary with each manufacturer. Table 9-1 is provided to acquaint you with some of the various properties of suture.

STORAGE OF SUTURE MATERIAL

Store all suture material in the same area, but segregate the various types to facilitate inventory and promote speedy selection:

1. Either by use (ophthalmic, cardiovascular, general closure, etc.)

2. Or by type (silk, surgical gut, synthetic, wire, etc.).

Whatever system of grouping is used, keep sizes in order (5-0, 4-0, etc.). Rotate material so that older suture will be used first. Be alert as to expiration dates.

When sutures are stored in each OR, and the box supply is low, it is not acceptable practice to "refill" from another box. It is not only a time waster and poor aseptic technique, but it also mixes up the "lot" numbers and expiration dates.

Note: Sutures, like suturing devices, are considered "medical devices," and are therefore controlled by the FDA. At the time of manufacture, the suture manufacturer imprints each box with a "lot" number. Thus, if any sutures are found to be defective, the manufacturer is able to trace and recall the particular lot.

Table 9-1
COMMONLY USED SUTURE MATERIAL

Name	Absorbable	Used When Infection Present	Desirable Features	Comments
Silk	No	No	Pliable Ends can be cut close to knot Does not dissolve prior to wound healing High tissue reaction	Loses tensile strength when exposed to moisture; is used dry
Plain surgical gut	Yes	Yes	Easily absorbed Minimal tissue reaction (but more than chromic)	Used especially for lesser vessels and in subcutaneous tissue
Chromic surgical gut	Yes	Yes	Slower absorption Minimal tissue reaction	Used to ligate larger vessels and suture deeper tissue
Nylon (monofilament)	No	No	High tensile strength Permits uniform approximation	Needs special knotting procedure

Surgical steel (wire)	No	Yes	High tensile strength Nonirritating to tissue	Popularly used in plastic and ophthalmic surgery, and microsurgery Difficult to tie Often used in orthopedics
Polyglactin 910 (Vicryl) Polyglycolic acid (Dexon)	Yes	Yes	High tensile strength Absorbed by hydrolysis in tissue	Holds tensile strength for 21 to 28 days Not subject to premature absorption (as can occur with chromic) due to patient's condition (e.g., infection, debilitation)
Polypropylene (Prolene, Surgilene)	No	Yes	Low tissue reaction Knot security	Popular for plastic and cardiovascular surgery
Polydioxanone (PDS)	Yes	Yes	Minimal tissue reaction Knot security	Retains strength longer than other synthetic materials

BASIC CONSIDERATIONS

The following considerations should be applied to the care and handling of suture material:

1. Examine the outer wrap of the packet for hole or defect.

2. Open the peel-away wrap carefully to prevent contamination of the inner packet.

3. Open only the amount you need.

4. Save unused, clean inner packets. Manufacturers will usually reprocess the suture.

5. At surgical field, note the immediate return of plastic reels (avoids possible loss in wound).

6. Remember, needled sutures must be counted.

7. Do not open sutures too far in advance. Long exposure to air can dry surgical gut.

8. At operative field, hold the suture packet at the border, tear along the dotted line, and in a direction *away from the operative wound*. Careless pressure on the center of a gut packet containing fluid (usually alcohol and water) will squirt the solution into the wound or into your eyes.

9. Dragging your fingers tightly along the surgical gut strand, or careless handling in the suture towel, tends to fray the fibers and weaken the suture. Clamping any suture tends to weaken it at that point.

10. Avoid pulling surgical gut. To straighten it, gently let the surgical gut slip through your hand, and then pull gently.

11. After passing a suture to the surgeon, have a scissors or clamp ready for his use.

12. The length of the suture depends on the depth and accessibility.

13. Have regard for cleanliness of the room. Do not throw used strands or packets on the floor.

14. Always know what size suture you are handling. Keep each size separate. Standardize locations of materials. *Habit pattern* prevents confusion and increases your speed. Be sure the surgeon knows what size or type of suture you are giving him.

In selecting sutures, there is no hard-and-fast rule to follow. The preceding information, correlated with the type of body tissue and its condition, determines the type and size of suture selected. *For example:*

1. The suture material needed to tie the cystic artery (a large vessel) must be strong, and ought not to be absorbed before the vessel is securely sealed. Chromic surgical gut has that quality. The surgeon is working in a deep cavity, so your suture must be long and be able to withstand considerable pull. Size 0 or 1 chromic in half length would answer those needs.

2. A patient may have a recurrent hernia. The surgeon may request wire, or another strong, nonabsorbable suture or mesh in view of this repeated hernia.

For practice, think of a particular operation. Attempt to determine the sizes and types of sutures required by the tissue involved, vessels encountered, etc.

SUTURING DEVICES

Whereas "regular" suture material is used during an operation, there are times when a suturing device satisfactorily facilitates a step in the procedure. It also decreases the length of time formerly required for the operation.

The devices range in design and are constantly undergoing improvement for ease of operation. Types of suturing devices, and their functions, are listed below.

1. Suturing devices often referred to as "staple guns" are made in various sizes and configurations for particular anatomical structures. When properly placed and activated, they "fire" a row of staples for ligation or anastomosis. In other words, it is an automatic suture. Basic considerations regarding the use of the "staple gun" are:
   a. The staples for such are supplied in small racks designed to fit the gun.
   b. It is imperative that the nurse know how to assemble the instrument (particularly if it has component parts), select the correct size staples, and load the gun.
   c. It is, obviously, also essential that the nurse know how to clean and reload the gun.
   d. The staples are expensive and are often a patient charge.

2. Vessels and small structures can be ligated by use of ligating clips. They are used in place of free suture ties or suture ligatures for control of hemostasis. Important considerations include the following:
   a. The appliers are of various lengths and widths to accommodate the anatomical location and the size of the different clips.

   b. The technique of loading the applier, though basically simple, must be learned.
   c. Care must be used in transferring the loaded applier to the surgeon.

3. Skin closure devices, often called "skin staplers," are popular because one can rapidly close the skin with acceptable cosmetic results. The staplers of various manufacturers are preloaded, and differ in design, ability, and size of staples used, to suit a particular need (e.g., a cosmetic facial procedure requires smaller staples than does an abdominal incision).
   a. The stapler is prepackaged sterile and is disposable—so to prevent waste, select the proper, requested size.
   b. Staple removers are also available, and although rarely used in the OR, a few should be available.

   Each surgeon's ideas on the subjects of suture material and suturing devices have been formulated by training, experience, and research. Preferences will vary, but the surgeon's choice is founded on principles. A nurse must adapt to the variations in practice.

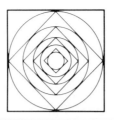

Chapter 10

Suture Needles

Needles are used for the placement of sutures. Selection of needles for surgery depends upon the type of tissue involved, the approach to the area— whether intricate or accessible— and the personal preference of the surgeon.

Today, the use of "free" needles is rare because of the availability of swaged sutures (needles are attached to the suture at the time of manufacture). Not only is the latter convenient for use, but it also affords the surgeon a wide variety of needle shapes and sizes that are best suited for the anatomical structure and the surgical procedure.

However, it is important for you to be aware of what is available. *For example:*

1. Note the variety of swaged suture needles. (Notice that very fine sutures have very fine needles.)

2. Observe the "free" needles that are available. Most hospitals buy sterile disposable needles because of

convenience, assurance of sharpness, and sterility readiness.

There are three parts to a needle: eye, body, and point. Any of these parts may vary in design to adapt the needle to a particular tissue, or to serve a special purpose.

THE EYE

The eye of the suture needle may vary in size, shape, or configuration, or may not even be present.

1. Eyed needle
   a. Shape of the eye aids in identifying the needle, and suggests its use. (A thin, oblong eye is found on intestinal needles; a needle designed for fascia or muscle usually has a heavy, rectangular eye.)
   b. Size of the eye must conform to the diameter of the suture material.
   - *Narrow eye*—designed to accept fine-gauge suture. The diameter of the suture material must not be larger than the diameter of the eye. This prevents fraying of suture material.
   - *Wider rectangular eye*—designed to accommodate larger-gauge suture material. Do not use this type with fine-gauge suture material, as it would result in unnecessary tissue trauma.

2. Split eye (French eye) needle
   On close observation you will note that the eye is actually two fine prongs (split at the end). Surgeons prefer this type of needle for suturing with fine silk in intestinal work, as it is less traumatic in results— more like a fused or swaged needle.

3. Swaged needle (referred to as *atraumatic* needle) Suture material is fused, or swaged, to the needle. There is no eye. Important factors are:
   a. The diameter of the suture is about the same as that of the needle—thus there is less trauma to tissue.
   b. The needle and suture are ready for use—thus it is a time-saver.

THE BODY

The body (or shaft) is the main portion of the needle. Consider the following variations:

1. The body may be straight or curved. The curves may form ½ of a circle, ⅜ of a circle, etc.

2. The body may be round or have a cutting edge.

3. The body may taper from a larger diameter to a smaller diameter.

THE POINT

This is the tip of the needle. Types of points include:

1. *Taper point*—the body of the needle, from its largest diameter, gradually tapers to a sharp point.

2. *Blunt point*—designed to pass sutures around vascular or poorly exposed areas.

3. *Trocar point*—triangular cutting-edged point. The trocar point is:
   a. Easily passed through tough tissue.
   b. Not used on friable tissue.

USE OF A NEEDLE HOLDER
WITH THE NEEDLE

A needle holder is an instrument used to hold the suture needle firmly in place for suturing. To adapt to the suture area and needle design, needle holders are made in various patterns of weight, length, and tip construction.

To choose the location of hold on the needle, use the following as a guide:

1. If the holder is placed on or too close to the eye or the swaged end (a weak part of the needle), the needle may possibly break.

2. If the holder is placed too far down the shaft, you limit the passage of the needle through the tissue, causing a delay in suturing.

3. Place the holder a little below the eye or swaged end, allowing about three-quarters of the needle to remain free.

4. Place the needle near the tip of the holder to facilitate suturing.

To choose the correct needle holder:

1. When a fine needle is required for intricate work, use a needle holder with a lighter-pattern tip (rather than one with a heavy design). A heavy-design tip will bend or possibly break the fine needle.

2. When a heavy needle is required, use a needle holder with a heavy-pattern tip (rather than one with a delicate design). A delicate-design tip will be "sprung" by the heavy needle, and will no longer be able to hold a fine needle securely.

Table 10-1
THREADING A SUTURE NEEDLE

Procedure	*Purpose*
Eyed needle	
Thread from the inner curvature to the outer curvature.	The needle is less likely to become unthreaded, as there is less stress on the outer curvature.
Determine the length of the short end or "tail" of the suture. Observe the surgeon's use of suture.	Suturing in deep, inaccessible areas requires a longer "tail" (approx. 4 inches). But when suturing in exposed areas, using interrupted sutures, 2 inches is usually sufficient.
If the needle is difficult to thread, cut the suture end diagonally.	This provides a point that will slip into the needle eye.
French eye needle	
Thread by holding the short end of the suture under tension and pressing the side of the strand between the prongs.	If threaded at the center instead of the short end, the prongs may fray the suture material and weaken it.
Determine the length of the short end of the suture.	Same as for an eyed needle.
Check prongs for working order.	Constant placing of suture material into the eye tends to weaken the prongs.

THREADING A SUTURE NEEDLE

To determine the correct procedure for threading a suture needle, refer to Table 10-1.

BASIC CONSIDERATIONS

Some basic considerations regarding the use of suture needles are as follows:

1. Do not use defective needles.
   a. Points are dulled by use. Curves become distorted by hard use.
   b. Inspect for nicks, burrs, and corrosion.
   c. Inspect a swaged suture for weakness at the point of fusion with the needle.

2. Keep an accurate count of needles at all times (before the case starts, during the case as swaged needle sutures are added for procedure, and at the end of the case). The count must tally (see Chapter 11).

3. Follow your OR's procedure for placement of used needles (e.g., on magnetic holder, in packet).

4. Inquire of your supervisor as to what is done in the event a needle is lost or a count is incorrect (e.g., search procedure, X-ray, incident report).

5. Always see to the *immediate return* of the needle (this holds for the eyed, i.e., free, and swaged types) for the following reasons:
   a. Prompt recognition of loss is repaid by prompt recovery of the needle.
   b. Assuring immediate return of the needle avoids complicated search (in the wound, or on the table or floor).

6. Free needles, when not on needle holders, must be securely located in a specific area. Doing so:
   a. Prevents accidental sweeping of needles into the operative wound.
   b. Speeds handling because of the definite placement of needles.

7. Always have at least two needles of the same type on setup. It prevents time loss while suturing.

8. When a needle pricks a glove, discard the needle and change the glove.

9. Have the circulating nurse pick up needles that drop to the floor. Accurate check for a lost needle is impossible when a room may have a needle from a preceding case on the floor.

10. Needles used on the septic part of a case should not be used for closure of a wound. *For example:*
    a. Total hysterectomy—vaginal vault needles are considered contaminated.
    b. Intestinal suturing—needles used on mucosa are considered contaminated.

CARE AND STORAGE OF
FREE NONDISPOSABLE NEEDLES

Observe the following procedures regarding the care and storage of free nondisposable needles:

1. Assure that needles are clean and free from tissue and blood prior to sterilization.

2. Sterilize needles before and after use, in order to:
   a. Protect the patient.
   b. Protect the person handling needles after the operation.

3. Store needles in a dry place to prevent rust.

4. Store needles of the same type and size together. Segregation:
   a. Speeds selection.
   b. Facilitates inventory.

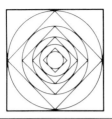

Chapter 11

Counts

The surgical wound and the patient's body must not be subjected to the presence of foreign bodies, unless, of course, the foreign object is meant to be there (e.g., vessel clip, prosthesis). The performance of surgery requires the use of instruments, sponges, needles, etc., within the body—on a temporary basis. Because such objects are temporary, they must be removed (retrieved) before the closure of the wound. To confirm retrieval, "counts" are essentially done.

You must learn the established count system of your OR. Your integrity is vital.

GUIDELINES

The following guidelines are provided to acquaint you with a general system of counts.

1. A "count sheet" is used to record the number (amounts) of each item. Items (other than instru-

ments) are listed according to their packaged amounts. *For example:*

```
4 × 4 sponges  −  10 + 10 + 10
lg. lap pads   −   5 + 5
peanuts        −   5
```

2. Retrieved items are collected in similar groups and items crossed off (slash mark). For example, when ten 4 × 4 sponges have been collected, it would be indicated as follows:

```
4 × 4 sponges  −  1̶0̶ + 10 + 10
```

3. Discarded items should be picked up immediately to prevent loss.

4. Small items (e.g., peanut sponges) should not be discarded in a bucket "one at a time." They can be easily overlooked by the circulating nurse. Rather, collect a group (packaged amount) and then discard.

5. Items to be counted include instruments, sponges, lap pads, umbilical tape, vessel loops, removable clamp protectors, needles, and cottonoids. (Future advanced products may well be added to the list.)

6. Counts are done simultaneously by the circulating nurse and scrub nurse (scrub assistant).

7. Counts are done before the surgical procedure is started.

8. As countable items are delivered to the field throughout the procedure, the scrub nurse counts the items (witnessed by the circulating nurse), and they are recorded.

9. Counts are checked for the proper tally before any cavity is closed (e.g., uterus, as in a cesarean section), as well as at the final cavity closure.

10. Counts are checked again before the skin closure.

11. When personnel relieve one another (e.g., for lunch break), counts are checked. That places the responsibility on the proper person and reduces future problems or conflicts.

12. Countable items must never leave the room until after the patient leaves—there might be a future problem. Refer to your supervisor for the rule.

13. At the time of final tally, the scrub nurse reports verbally to the surgeon. (This is done at each cavity closure, as well as at the pre-skin closure.)

14. A note is made on the chart (or OR record)—stating the condition of the final count—and signed by both the scrub nurse and circulating nurse.

15. When the count does not tally:
    a. Report it immediately to the surgeon.
    b. A search of the wound and room (including hampers) is done.
    c. If the item is not found, summon assistance to help with the room search. Alert the supervisor.

16. If the item is not retrieved:
    a. Follow hospital policy.
    b. Write up an inciaent report.

Note: Hospital procedure usually mandates an immediate X-ray. You then record the findings on the incident report. Physicians and personnel must follow the policy.

The question often arises as to what cases require counts. It is safe practice to do counts on all cases, but it depends on hospital policy. Be aware that sponges have been lost in a bunionectomy procedure, and litigation ensued. The advantages of counting on all cases are that:

1. It ensures that patient, physician, nurse, and hospital are protected.

2. Instrument sets stay complete (prevents unnoticed loss of instrument in hamper).

If setups are organized, count sheets are simplified and workable, and the nurse team is efficient and co-operative, the count procedure can be done quickly and accurately—and will not provoke the wrath of the surgeon.

Everyone must realize the importance of counts. The supervisor and the chief of surgery should be made aware of any negative attitudes.

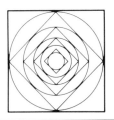

Chapter 12

Positioning the Patient

There are specific positions in which the patient must be placed so that the desired surgery can be performed. Each type of operation has its individual demands, and so has each patient. The positioning procedures are patterned to best fulfill those requirements. Improper positioning necessitates the moving of the patient during procedures. That means time loss and the possibility of contamination.

PREPARING THE OPERATING ROOM

Have all accessories (braces, pillows, footboard, straps, leg holders, etc.) for the desired position in readiness and conveniently located. Doing so:

1. Conserves time.

2. Prevents the nurse from leaving the patient and anesthesiologist to get extra equipment.

3. Expedites the procedure to the satisfaction of the surgeon and anesthesiologist.

4. Maintains aseptic technique.
   a. Accessories hurriedly brought into the operating room may not be clean.
   b. Accessories must be placed a safe distance from the sterile setup.

5. Prevents confusion.
   a. The room is quiet; therefore, emotional trauma to the patient is not increased.
   b. Handling of the patient is minimized.
   c. The task is done with assurance.

Have the operating room table properly located and *locked*, as follows:

1. Allow sufficient room on all sides of the table for entrance of the patient and for transfer (this prevents contamination).

2. Confirm the position of the table in proper relation to the overhead spotlight, microscope, or other overhead fixed apparatus (e.g., X-ray).

3. Lock the table in place to prevent injury to the patient in transfer from the stretcher or bed to the OR table.

TRANSFERRING THE PATIENT TO THE OPERATING ROOM TABLE

A nurse and a co-worker must be in attendance when transferring a patient to the operating room table. Place the stretcher next to the locked table. One person stands at the side of the stretcher, holding it closely

against the table; the other person stands on the opposite side of the operating room table, ready to receive
the patient. That prevents the patient from falling between the stretcher and the table, and from falling off
the far side of the table.

Proper regard must be given to the patient's needs
during transfer. *For example:*

1. Provide steady traction for a fracture, if needed.

2. Guard against the accidental removal of tubes or
   catheters, IVs, or monitor leads.

3. If the patient is obese, guard against possible tip-
   ping of the stretcher. Exert downward pressure on
   your side of the stretcher as the patient shifts his
   weight to the opposite side.

4. Always consider the patient's comfort *and* security.

5. Always consider the patient's emotional needs (e.g.,
   refer to the OR table as the OR "bed," as in "We are
   transferring you to the OR bed").

PLACING THE PATIENT
IN CORRECT POSITION

There are *four* main points to consider when placing
patients in position for surgery: *anatomy, comfort,
safety,* and *respiratory freedom.* The use of local or general anesthesia does not alter those four main points.
Many institutions have certain positions established
for operative procedures. They will be referred to as
"kidney position," "chest position," "lithotomy position," etc. When those established positions are used
as intended by their originators, anatomy, comfort,

safety, and respiratory freedom of the patient have been taken care of.

Danger is present when the positions are not interpreted correctly, or when you devise the proper patient position yourself. To eliminate that danger, let the four points be your guide.

ANATOMY INVOLVED

Be aware of the following with respect to anatomy:

1. Know the location of the area to be treated. *For example:*
   a. Location of organs or tumors.
   b. Right or left extremity.
   c. Area to be skin grafted, etc.

2. Know the surgeon's approach and preferences:
   a. There is more than one established position for many procedures.
   b. The operative area must be easily accessible.
   c. The surgeon should assist, and confirm that the anatomical position is correct.

COMFORT

Assure the patient's comfort at all times.

1. The patient must be in a comfortable position, whether conscious or unconscious. When the patient is conscious, it is tiring for him to hold the required position. When the patient is unconscious, beware of placing him in a position that is not anatomically normal.

a. Support the head, body, and extremities.
b. Prevent postoperative muscular discomfort or paralysis by guarding against:

- Arms extended and placed above shoulder level.
- Shoulder braces over brachial nerve sites.
- Hands clenched and placed too far under buttocks during surgery.
- Incorrect practice of lifting one leg at a time for lithotomy position (same is true when returning patient to dorsal recumbent position).
- Inadequate support of the hips in lithotomy position.
- Legs crossed during the anesthesia period.
- Portable instrument stand touching toes.
- Feet hanging off the table.

2. Do not expose the patient unnecessarily.
   a. Embarrassment is present for the conscious patient.
   b. Professional code dictates respect for an unconscious patient.

SAFETY

Ensure that proper safety precautions are taken:

1. Safeguard the point of entry of intravenous.
   a. Do not interrupt the flow of necessary intravenous fluids.
   b. Avoid infiltration of fluids into soft tissue.

2. Protect body areas from injury. *For example:*
   a. Give special regard to body parts, e.g., fingers—be sure they will not be caught in a table "break."

 b. Cover sandbags, position supports, etc., with towels to prevent skin irritation.
 c. Protect the patient from pressure when using footboard, lateral supports, head brace, or perineal post. (The area or article may have to be padded with a sheet, Webril, etc.)

3. Assure that equipment used for positioning is clean, to safeguard the patient against infection.

4. Safeguard the patient against falling.
 a. Apply the leg strap correctly, when its use is requested by the anesthesiologist or surgeon.
 b. Use table appliances or adhesive tape to ensure safe maintenance of position.

5. Restrain hands of conscious patients. (Explain to the patient the reasons for restraining his hands, and then restrain them in a comfortable position.) Doing so:
 a. Prevents the possibility that the wound may become contaminated.
 b. Avoids unnecessary interruption of the surgical procedure.

6. Apply the cautery grounding pad after the patient is positioned, in order to:
 a. Avoid "tenting" of the pad.
 b. Allow for proper grounding.
 c. Prevent patient burns.

Note: *Be sure* you know the mechanical operation of the table, and the location of accessories and how they are used. Practice putting the table in various positions.

RESPIRATORY FREEDOM

In order to provide for respiratory freedom:

1. Relieve chest and abdominal areas from external pressure. *For example:*
   a. Prone positions. Support the rib cage with soft rolls, or use a specially designed mattress that allows for unrestrained chest expansion.
   b. Lithotomy positions. Obese patients or patients with respiratory limitations must not suffer additional respiratory embarrassment from the weight of an arm restrained over the chest area.
   c. Lateral positions. Elevate the rib cage from the operating table with a small resilient pad.

2. Aid in establishing an adequate respiratory airway by position. *For example:*
   a. For patients undergoing head and neck surgery, place a soft roll under the patient's shoulders to prevent flexion of the trachea.
   b. When applying dressings or body casts to anesthetized patients, hold the head in extended position to maintain a normal respiratory airway.

Remember: When the patient has been placed in position, and when you can say, "This patient is *comfortable*, necessary *safety* measures have been taken, *respiratory freedom* is established, and the *anatomy* for surgery has been considered," then you have provided optimum patient care.

TRANSFERRING THE PATIENT TO THE POST-ANESTHESIA STRETCHER

The same precautions and techniques are exercised here as in transferring the patient to the operating room table. However, more assistance is needed, as the patient is usually asleep and cannot help himself. Besides the necessity for personnel on either side of the OR bed, additional support is needed on either end. The transfer must be smooth. To ensure this:

1. Await the anesthesiologist's permission.

2. Do not lift the patient and "bounce" him onto the stretcher—it can induce shock.

3. Protect the surgical wound from injury, offering support of the area, limb, etc.

4. Prevent accidental removal of a Foley catheter, intravenous, or other tubes/drains.

5. Exercise care in transferring equipment (e.g., underwater seal apparatus—temporary clamping of tubes may be desired).

Prevent injury to personnel, as follows:

1. Summon additional help.

2. Use a special patient roller.

3. Use proper body mechanics when lifting.

Consider other patient needs before leaving the room. Provide the warmth of a blanket, use of side rails or straps, and a small arm board for the intravenous site. *Await the anesthesiologist's readiness before transferring the patient.*

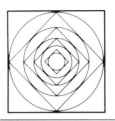

Chapter 13
Draping

The term "draping" is used in the OR to describe the covering of tables, stands, and the patient (leaving only the area for surgery exposed). Sterile towels, table covers, and drape sheets of various sizes or specific designs are employed to provide an aseptic area for the placement of sterile instruments and supplies, as well as an aseptic area for the surgical procedure. Skill and technique in handling these drapes must be mastered to preserve the fundamental purpose of their use. To achieve successful aseptic draping, the nurse must plan her work.

The OR is provided with a variety of sterile "set-up" packs. In addition to the basic table and stand covers, setup packs may contain other items such as surgical gowns, towels, patient drapes, etc. Some packs consist of only a single item such as a lithotomy drape, lap sheet, etc.; others are designed for use in specific procedures such as cystoscopy, arthroscopy, etc., and contain the articles that are necessary for the procedure.

DRAPING MATERIALS

The use of disposable nonwoven material has proved to be successful in affording a sterile field and in preventing breakthrough of liquids and body fluids. Basic considerations regarding the use of disposable nonwoven materials are:

1. They come prepackaged—designed for basic or specific OR procedures.

2. They require less room for storage.

3. They have eliminated many of the problems inherent in the use of linen (e.g., holes, labor in washing and processing).

4. They can be cost-effective (when compared with labor, inspection, and processing costs of linen).

5. They are not cost-effective if they are improperly selected and carelessly handled, and if wasteful use is not prevented.

Linen packs are used in some institutions. Important factors regarding their use are as follows:

1. Packs are designed for specific use.

2. The nurse must be alert in observing for defects such as holes, and must exercise care in preventing tears and holes.

3. Huck (a type of linen) towels are used in conjunction with disposable drapes, and serve an excellent purpose.

It is advantageous to spend time looking at the various draping packs and materials available in the OR. Manufacturers' catalogues depict pack contents and draping designs. If linen is used, observe the way materials are folded, the sterilization process, etc. It familiarizes the nurse with what supplies are available, what articles are contained in the packs and where located, and how certain sheets and towels are folded. The nurse who becomes aware of the labor and cost involved will be more careful in handling drapes, and less likely to waste supplies.

Know available draping material. *For example:*

1. Know the sizes of sheets. (Seeing the area to be draped or covered, you can visualize the size sheet or number of sheets you will need.)

2. Know the specifically designed drapes available. (They were made to afford exposure of a certain area for a particular operation.)

3. Know the drape configurations and how the drape is unfolded during the draping procedure. (This increases your skill in handling the drapes.)

Conform to the draping policies of the institution. *For example:*

1. Know the required padding for sterile instrument tables and stands. Double thickness is necessary when linen is used. The impervious nonwoven disposable drapes designed for table covers require a single thickness.

2. Know the required layers of sterile patient drapes for orthopedics, extremities, etc.

3. Know the variations in techniques used for ear, nose, throat, and eye procedures.

Select drapes designed to accomplish the task, or improvise intelligently. Prior to opening packages, estimate the tables, stand, microscope, or other equipment needed to be draped, and determine the type of drape required by the patient.

PREPARE THE OPERATING ROOM

In preparing the operating room, have only the necessary furniture in the room, in order to:

1. Provide more working area.

2. Reduce the possibility of contamination.

3. Eliminate potential obstructions to carrying out the procedure.

   Inspect furniture for the presence of dust, and remove it by using a cloth moistened with disinfectant. It prevents airborne contamination via dust particles.

   Remove moisture from furniture. Wet tables contaminate linen drapes and lessen the margin of safety for disposable drapes.

   Place furniture in the area of use whenever possible, for the following reasons:

1. It renders the area convenient for work, thereby saving time and motion.

2. The moving of draped objects increases the chance of contamination.

3. Accessibility saves time at the start of the surgical procedure. (Setup is organized and ready to go.)

PRINCIPLES OF DRAPING

Conform to *aseptic techniques*:

1. Protect hands from contamination when draping.

    a. The drape must shield gloved hands at all times.

    b. When placing the drape, lift your hands and keep them *well above* the unsterile area. (If you keep your hands down, you are likely to touch the unsterile area.)

2. Protect your gown from contamination, as follows:

    a. Do not reach across an unsterile area, as in passing a towel to a doctor on the other side of the undraped patient.

    b. Be constantly aware of unsterile areas, apparatus, people, etc., around you. *Remember*, your gown is loose-fitting; so you actually need more room than you would normally to prevent contact with objects.

3. *Place* sterile drapes; do not flip or toss them carelessly. You must have control of the drape, no matter how large. *For example:*

    a. Do not allow drapes to drag on the floor.

    b. Keep the drape away from the area below your waist and away from sides of furniture. (By giving yourself room to unfold the drape, and by keeping your arms extended from your body, you can avoid contamination of the drape.)

    c. Be sure you see all areas when you are draping. (This seems so simple; yet there have been many instances of contamination when a nurse has blindly wrapped a drape around a limb, or handled a large sterile sheet without being able to see over it.)

4. Remember that placed sterile drapes cannot be rearranged to achieve asepsis of an area. If the drape is not satisfactory, either have it removed or add an

extra drape to adequately cover the area. (By moving drapes to different positions, you contaminate the area.) For example: Suppose you have covered a sterile table and you notice the drape does not adequately cover one end, while the other end shows excess of drape. You cannot shift the drape. Below the table edge is considered unsafe, and you would be pulling a part of the drape that is of questionable sterility over an area that must be sterile.

5. As some drapes require two people to perform the task, wait for assistance. (This also refers to the placement of the available plastic-type material that is adhered to the prepared operative area and which takes the place of wound towels.)

6. Always check the drape pack for integrity of the wrapper.

7. Discard damp drapes and drapes with holes. (The field is not considered sterile if either of these is present.)

8. Read the sterility expiration date on the package. Observe the sterilization indicator located inside cloth packs. Do not use packs when sterilization is questionable.

9. Secure drapes in the desired position at the time of placement. It avoids:
   a. Shifting of the drape during the procedure.
   b. Unnecessary redraping during the procedure.
   c. Contamination that may go unrecognized.

Arrange drapes required to execute the entire patient drape in the order of use. Forethought and planning save time and motion. You:

1. Avoid omissions.

2. Prevent confusion.

3. Conserve anesthesia time.

   Include in the arrangement odd items such as:

1. Bandage to secure a towel about the hand or foot.

2. Required number of towel clips to secure the drape.

3. Fluffs to protect the perineum from antiseptic solutions when preparing adjacent areas.

   Exercise care when attending to the removal of drapes postoperatively.

1. Remove towel clips or other devices that secure the drape, in order to:
   a. Prevent injury to the patient.
   b. Prevent needless tearing of linen.

2. Shake drapes prior to placement in the appropriate hamper, in order to:
   a. Prevent loss of instruments.
   b. Prevent injury to laundry and housekeeping personnel.

   Draping requires forethought and practice. Your speed and safety will be increased if you spend some spare time practicing the opening of towels, unfolding and placing of sheets in position, and planning supplies required by specific cases. When practicing, it is helpful to put on a gown and gloves so that you accustom yourself to the added precautions needed in a real situation.

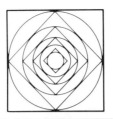

Chapter 14
Care of Specimens/ Cultures

When something is removed from a patient's body, it is usually referred to as a "specimen." It could be an organ, a sample of tissue, body fluid, or a foreign body. (A foreign body is anything that is not normally a part of the human structure, e.g., a prosthesis, an appliance, a piece of glass, a bullet.) The nurse is entrusted with the specimen handling, saving, and labeling, and the processing of laboratory forms. Consequently, attention to detail, including confirmation of delivery to the laboratory, is of the utmost importance.

MEDICAL REASONS

Medical reasons that require extreme care regarding specimens are:

1. The specimen may be very important for further diagnosis and treatment.

2. The specimen (body part) may be used subsequently for a transplant.

3. The hospital tissue committee reviews surgical cases to assess the quality of medical care being delivered.

4. Culture specimens are not only valuable for diagnosis, but may well be studied for antibiotic sensitivity, which assists in patient treatment.

LEGAL REASONS

Legal reasons include the following:

1. Specimens represent legal evidence that something (e.g., a gallbladder) was removed. A patient may allege that it was not done.

2. A foreign body such as a bullet is legal evidence, and may possibly be involved in a court case.

3. A foreign body such as an orthopedic plate with screws requires the documentation and count of each item (e.g., a specimen of a five-hole plate and four screws would indicate a screw was left in the body).

OTHER REASONS

It is not uncommon for the laboratory to require that all tissue be sent for examination (this would include normal bone and skin). A gross examination, rather than a microscopic analysis, is determined by the pathologist and hospital policy. Such a procedure:

1. Allows for examination and verification by the pathologist.

2. Protects both the patient and the physician.

3. Confirms hospital conformity to state and federal regulations.

4. Confirms compliance to the requests of surveying and accrediting agencies.

SPECIMENS

Specimens are not permitted to leave the OR without complete identification, proper labeling, and pertinent clinical data recorded on the pathology form, and without some means of verification by the surgeon. The following procedure must be followed:

1. Have a receptacle or towel ready to receive the specimen.

2. Assure proper identification of the specimen. (What is it? Is it "right" or "left"?) Keep multiple specimens separated.

3. Exercise special care with small specimens. Air tends to dry tissue quickly, and that changes the gross appearance. Unless otherwise directed, moisten the specimen with saline immediately.

4. Package or prepare the specimen for the laboratory, according to standard rules in your hospital.

5. Prevent errors by confirming that the necessary information is present and correct (i.e., the patient's name and identification number, name of specimen, surgeon's name, other clinical data) before the specimen is taken to the OR specimen collection area. *Write legibly.*

6. Assure compliance to department rules for documentation (i.e., patient's chart or OR record form).

7. Use the method set up in the OR for recording all specimens taken from the suite.

FROZEN SECTIONS

During surgery, there are times when an immediate identification of the type of tissue mass is required. One method employed is a laboratory "frozen section" examination—so termed because the tissue is subjected to an immediate freezing process. It allows the pathologist to literally slice a minutely thin piece (section) of the tissue and examine it microscopically. Thus, a report is quickly available.

The OR nurse's responsibilities at this time are as follows:

1. The pathology department should be alerted that a frozen section is contemplated.

2. At the time the tissue is in the process of being removed, the OR nurse must inform the control desk to call the pathologist.

3. The specimen for frozen section should be placed on a towel or in a receptacle and kept moist with saline. The specimen should not be sent to the pathologist on a "counted" sponge.

4. The specimen must be properly labeled, and the pathology form must accompany the specimen.

5. The pathologist must be informed as to whether the patient is awake or asleep. He reports his findings directly to the surgeon, either in person or over an

intercom. (Certainly, an awake patient's anxiety would be heightened if the report was overheard.)

6. To protect the patient, surgeon, and nurse from errors or misinterpretation, the nurse does not communicate a verbal report. If the pathologist cannot use an intercom or be physically present, a written report from him is delivered to the surgeon.

CULTURES

Body fluids or tissues require the same attention, care, and compliance with hospital and laboratory regulations as specimens.

Cultures *must* be delivered to the laboratory promptly, for the following reasons:

1. Bacteria tend to multiply continually (e.g., a urine culture allowed to stand for a long period of time will show an increase in the number of bacteria present—hence, a report may give an untrue picture of the patient's condition).

2. Some laboratory tests require inoculation of various culture media, certain temperature climates, and a period of time for growth and identification. Patient treatment may be delayed unnecessarily.

Cultures must be accompanied by the proper laboratory form. Important points to keep in mind are:

1. There are designated forms for requested tests.

2. Careless marking of the form will result in loss of time for the laboratory and unnecessary charges to the patient.

3. Refer to the supervisor, laboratory authority, or laboratory procedure book for any needed clarification of procedure.

When cultures are requested for tissue or body fluids:

1. Have ready proper applicators, tubes, or containers (aerobic, anaerobic, specimen collector).

2. List the required information on the tube or container, and attach the proper laboratory slip.

3. Use the method for recording all cultures taken from the OR.

4. Assure the safe and immediate delivery of the culture to the laboratory, and be aware of the delivery procedure for all hours (day, evening, night).

OTHER BASIC CONSIDERATIONS

In addition to the above, the following considerations apply to cases involving specimens and cultures:

1. To prevent conflicts with the laboratory as to whether a specimen/culture was sent, follow the OR method of documentation of transfers.

2. In cases where legal evidence is crucial, as in those involving a bullet, be sure you know the proper procedure to be followed. Document actions taken.

3. In cases where a patient requests that the specimen be given to him (e.g., gallstones, bone plate), follow hospital rules. The specimen still must go to the laboratory for identification, but a notation such as "save for patient" can be indicated on the pathology form.

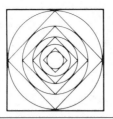

Chapter 15
The Mental Lineup

Prior to starting a procedure, you must *assemble yourself mentally*. This process should be going on well before you get to the field of operation. Preparing the sterile setup is only half the story.

Read your case assignment and take time to *think*. Do you know. . .

1. The anatomy involved?

2. The approach of the operating surgeon?

3. The approved technique of the hospital?

4. The professional capabilities of the nurse you are working with?

5. The general condition of the patient?

6. The emergencies brought about by the procedure?

Knowledge of those six points equips you for every type of surgery—from minor incision and drainage or change of dressing to complicated and lengthy procedures. The result of this "mental lineup" is that you conserve time, eliminate last-minute running, establish the doctor's confidence in you, and help achieve the ultimate goal—optimum patient care. Those six points concern the scrub nurse and the circulating nurse. Both must think along those lines. Each must be aware of the total situation and be prepared to assist the other.

ANATOMY INVOLVED

Basic anatomy must be understood to carry out any nursing procedure; in the operating room, it must be mastered. Knowledge of anatomy is the key to your success. Which instruments, drugs, sutures, sterile supplies, and extra equipment are required is partially determined by anatomical considerations. Before an operation, take time to consider the anatomy involved, and to anticipate and assess the problems that are present when dealing with specific structures. *For example:*

Pneumonectomy. Positioning the patient for surgery is dependent upon anatomy. Pneumonectomy requires the patient to be on his side. Thus, you need to have the proper supports to achieve that position, and to prevent pressure areas. The lungs lie within the rib cage; so you realize that a rib, or ribs, will have to be removed before the pertinent area of surgery can be exposed. For rib resection and retraction, special bone instruments must be added to the set. You visualize the attachment of the lung to the bronchus and the vascular supply of the lung; consequently, to cope with the depth and position, you add long instruments with particular angles, and you are reminded that sutures must be long, and needles of fine caliber, for delicate areas. Staple guns may be used to close the large bronchus, or in resecting lung tissue. A negative pressure exists within the chest cavity; when the chest is opened, that is destroyed. Therefore, after certain types of lung surgery are concluded, the negative pressure must be reestablished—a reminder to you of special tubes or drains to connect with an underwater seal.

The following examples list only one highlight. Think of the other considerations for each case.

Mastectomy.   The procedure involves a very vascular area; so have many extra clamps on hand.

Hysterectomy.   Ligation of uterine vessels is necessary. A curved clamp is desirable in view of the anatomical location.

Bone plating.   Select plates, screws, and bone-holding forceps in relation to the bone involved. For the same procedure, a fractured femur and a fractured humerus would require instruments of different sizes.

Eye work.   The eye structures are so small and delicate that the tiny instruments must be minutely examined for the presence of burrs or defects.

APPROACH OF THE SURGEON

Each surgeon has his own method of doing a routine procedure. Learn his method, so that you will be an efficient assistant. *For example:*

1. Have the surgeon's favorite instruments in the set-up. Many surgeons use instruments they bought themselves, and want them included in each case.

2. Have the sutures the surgeon prefers.

3. Does he desire a microscope? Image intensifier?

4. Will the surgeon desire the use of electric cautery?

5. What patient position does the surgeon request?

6. Will the surgeon drain through a stab wound or the incision?

APPROVED HOSPITAL TECHNIQUE

You must familiarize yourself with the approved technique as quickly as you can. You will learn the standards from the operating room supervisor, the senior nurse, and the operating room precedent book. Those standards have been devised by the medical board, staff doctors, operating room committee, and nursing supervisors to assure that approved and excellent patient care is rendered. You must do your part to maintain those institutional standards. Examples of some hospital policies are:

1. *Cancer technique.* Use a clamp once; then have it washed and resterilized.

2. *Orthopedics.* Use of double-glove technique for skin incision.

3. *Lost sponge or broken needle.* X-ray of the patient is required, and an incident report sheet must be filled out.

4. *Instrument, sponge, pad, and needle count.* Hospital-approved method.

5. *Drapes and operative skin preparations.* Hospital-approved method.

6. *Sterilization.*   The method (steam, ethylene oxide sterilization, or chemical disinfection) and the time required.

7. *Operative permits.*   Proper forms must be signed, witnessed, and dated.

8. *Septic or contaminated cases.*   The hospital may treat all cases as contaminated, but you must apply basic knowledge of bacteriology while carrying out nursing duties. Care for cultures per laboratory policy. Eliminate cross-contamination at all times, and protect your own well-being.

PROFESSIONAL CAPABILITIES
OF NURSES ON TEAM

Each team member is dependent upon the other team members for smooth execution of the operation. Time and many anxious moments are saved when you are aware of the other person's capabilities. You are then prepared to foresee or remedy a situation through supervision of operating room techniques and skills. Consider the following:

1. Is the nurse you are working with familiar with the procedure and general course of the operation?

2. Does she understand the importance and system of taking all the counts?

3. Does she know where the emergency equipment is kept, and how to use it or prepare it for use?

4. Is she aware of her responsibilities to the patient, surgeon, anesthesiologist, and scrub nurse?

5. Will it be necessary to have an additional person present to aid this nurse, so that her participation

will be a learning experience, but not at the expense of optimum patient care?

CONDITION OF THE PATIENT

The patient's condition affects every situation. There are "routine" methods used in setting up an operating room, but there is never a "routine" patient. Various considerations are:

1. *Emergency work*, such as accidents and acute illnesses (ectopic pregnancy, aortic aneurysm, perforated ulcer, evisceration), requires rapidity in setting up the operating room.

2. *Obesity* requires that additional instruments be ready on the tray. The presence of excessive fat necessitates the use of broader and deeper retractors for exposure, and of long-handled instruments to reach underlying structures.

3. *Poor operative risks* (e.g., cardiacs, asthmatics, infants, elderly persons, alcoholics) require supplementary OR preparation: available "crash cart"; resuscitative equipment; additional nurse power to meet the requests of the surgeon and anesthesiologist; warming apparatus to maintain body heat.

4. *Apprehensive patients* require understanding and constant reassurance. Always remember, *no patient should be left unattended in an operating room.*

5. *Preparation for postoperative care* requires that the recovery room, ICU, or nursing unit be notified when special equipment is needed (e.g., fracture bed, suction, oxygen, hypothermia unit, ventilators, monitoring equipment).

EMERGENCIES BROUGHT ABOUT
BY OPERATION

Every procedure in an operating room has the potential for emergency. Analyze each circumstance, and remember that "emergency" means something other than hemorrhage. *For example:*

1. A thyroidectomy may require a tracheotomy if tracheal obstruction or compression occurs.

2. Nasal fractures may require a Caldwell-Luc operation because of bone fragments in the antrum.

3. Dental cases need two suction setups. Bone fragments may plug one suction, so another must be available to guard the patient against the possibility of aspiration.

4. Patients under local anesthesia must be observed for adverse reaction to the drug, e.g., profuse diaphoresis, tremor, syncope, thready pulse, change in blood pressure.

5. An inflamed appendix may rupture during removal and contaminate the field.

6. During a dilatation and curettage, the uterus may be perforated, and an abdominal operation may be necessary.

7. As an infant's life may depend upon the mechanical establishment of respirations, always check the resuscitation apparatus before a cesarean section is performed.

8. Patients in prone position under anesthesia depress their respirations by their own body weight. Correct positioning helps reduce the surgical risk.

A "mental lineup" is essential in preparation for scrubbing or circulating for a surgical procedure. It is actually "logical forethought." The next chapter, "The Four-Clue System," takes the Mental Lineup and puts it into practice.

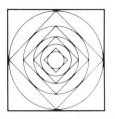

Chapter 16
The Four-Clue System

We have now reached a point at which we should refer concisely to operating room *procedure*. It is impossible to teach anyone every single step of every operative procedure (there are hundreds) and every possible deviation from routine in each procedure. What you will have to do, before you "scrub" for a case, is to study the operation, by reference to surgical books and conference notes, and to develop a method of thinking that prepares you for deviations in routine, new procedures, and complications that may arise.

The foregoing chapters described the overall operating room picture. Now let us concentrate on solving the procedure, from the selection of instruments to the application of the dressing. There are *four clues* that will help you solve the problem and make you a secure member of the surgical team. The clues must be used in the sequence given. As you proceed, visualize each answer.

Clue 1. Surgical approach
How will the area involved in the procedure be exposed? Ask yourself what position will be necessary to reach the operative area, how position will be maintained, what must be done before, for example, the appendix is removed, or the dilatation and curettage is performed.

Clue 2. Surgical procedure
The area is now exposed. What are the steps of the procedure at the operative site? What will you need to do during this phase?

Clue 3. Surgical complications
Ask yourself what unforeseen difficulties may possibly arise at the operative area that would require additional sutures, setups, or special equipment. What will you need to do to prepare for the various surgical complications?

Clue 4. Surgical closure
Anatomical layers are to be closed; dressings are to be applied. Ask yourself how the wound is to be closed and dressed. What will you need for the surgical closure?

Two examples in the use of the Four-Clue System are provided in Table 16-1. The descriptions are not complete from a surgical standpoint, nor are they intended to teach surgical nursing; rather, their purpose is to inspire logical thinking.

Table 16-1
APPLICATION OF THE FOUR-CLUE SYSTEM

Diagnostic Dilatation and Curettage

Clue	What you will need
1. Surgical approach (before the cervix is dilated and the uterus curetted)	
Patient in lithotomy position	Stirrups attached to table
Vaginal preparation	Receptacle, prep solution set
Bladder catheterized	Catheterization set
Patient draped	Specifically designed drape
Vagina retracted, cervix grasped	Instruments (vaginal retractor, tenaculum)
2. Surgical procedure	
Cervical os identified	Retractors, sponge stick
Uterus measured (depth)	Uterine sound
Cervix dilated	Complete set of dilators (small to large)
Uterus and cervix curetted	Opened sponge or Telfa pad to receive specimen; sharp and dull curettes of various sizes
Curettings collected	Sponge or Telfa pad with specimen carefully received
3. Surgical complications	
Cervical tear	Forceps, needle holder, suture, scissors, Kelly clamp, sponges
Perforation of uterus	If abdominal operation is requested, have setup available.
4. Surgical closure	
Sponge vaginal vault.	Sponges and sponge sticks
Apply perineal pad and cleanse adjacent area.	Perineal pad, moist towel

Continued

Table 16-1 *continued*

Pyloromyotomy (as done for congenital hypertrophic pyloric stenosis)

Clue	What you will need
1. Surgical approach	
Maintain body heat.	Overhead heating apparatus and/or thermal warming blanket; Webril-wrapped extremities
Dorsal recumbent position	Shorten OR bed (drop foot piece).
Infant secured to table	Tape or sheets
Surgical skin preparation	Skin prep solution set (warmed)
Drape	Towels, Steri-drape, or special drape
Abdominal incision, subcutaneous bleeders clamped	Knife, scissors, forceps, clamps (all of delicate design); sponges (counted); ligatures
Skin towels applied (if used)	Skin towels (small pads—counted); towel clamps
Peritoneal cavity opened and stomach exposed	Clean knife, thumb forceps, scissors, clamps and Babcock clamp in readiness, retractors
2. Surgical procedure	
Stomach grasped near pyloric ring and delivered into open wound; examined	Small moist pad, Babcock clamp
Incision into hypertrophied muscle	Delicate knife blade, sponge stick
Muscle fibers separated until mucosa pouts through	Small curved clamp
3. Surgical complications	
Accidental incision into duodenum	Suture for closure, or to hold omental patch. Gastric tube will be passed and attached to suction.

Clue	What you will need
4. Surgical closure	
Edges of peritoneum grasped	Clamps; instrument, sponge, pad, and needle count
Peritoneum closed	Forceps, needle holder, suture, scissors, and sponge stick
Muscle and fascia sutured	Forceps, sutures, scissors
Skin towels (if used) or Steri-drape removed from skin edge	Receive towels in receptacle; recheck counts.
Skin edges approximated	Forceps, suturing device, or skin sutures and scissors
Dressing or collodion applied	Gauze, tape, or collodion

The following example is a simple procedure, in comparison with others, but one that must be performed within a limited anesthesia period. The clues will be listed; can you supply the needs?

Change of Burn Dressing

Clue 1. **Surgical approach** *(What will you need to do the following?)*

   a. Remove old dressings.

   b. Place the old dressings in the designated receptacle.

   c. Cover exposed burned areas with sterile towels or sheets.

Clue 2. **Surgical procedure** *(What will you need to do the following?)*

   a. Remove sterile towels or sheets from the area to be treated.

   b. Remove decayed tissue.

   c. Clean off drainage that has formed on good tissue. Skin graft may be desired.

Clue 3. Surgical complications *(Can you meet these added surgical needs?)*
a. Infection (the presence of a pathogenic organism).
b. Shock.

Clue 4. Surgical closure *(Are the needed materials in readiness?)*
a. Special moist or medicated dressings must be applied.
b. Pressure dressing may be used (e.g., elastic bandages, Kerlix).

Now check whether you thought of these needs:

1. The surgical pack or packets to set up the sterile table (sheets, drapes, towels, sponges, gloves, gowns, basins, prep equipment)

2. Plastic bags for soiled dressings and for disposal of decayed tissue

3. Laundry bag

4. Sterile saline for irrigation and for moistening of skin grafts (possibly asepto syringe and suction)

5. Instruments (knife, scissors, forceps, short hemostats, sponge sticks, delicate-design needle holders, towel clamps)

6. Fine sutures or suturing device for skin graft

7. Skin graft setup and an extra table for same; dermatome and blade; lubricant for skin and applicator to apply; also knife, forceps, clamp, scissors, skin mesher, saline, and sponges

8. Culture tubes and labels.

Have you also anticipated these needs?

1. Did you remember the location of the crash cart?

2. Did you have special burn packs, bandage, and dressings on hand?

3. Did you request extra nurse power to support the patient in transfer, support a limb, assist the anesthesiologist, or assist with an emergency measure?

4. Did you remember the proper care of equipment and terminal disinfection of it and the room?

The example above and the two provided in Table 16-1 show you the way of logical thinking and its value in the operating room. The Four-Clue System is a structured process (framework) that enables you to anticipate and prepare in advance the needs for a surgical procedure, including potential complications. It is a matter of thinking of "first things first" and preventing you from becoming "lost." Remember, the individual needs of the patient must be incorporated into any plan of care.

For practice, select another procedure, and visualize what you will need for each of the *four clues*.

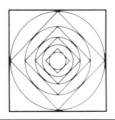

Chapter 17

Responsibility to the Anesthesiologist

Although the activity of the staff is concentrated on the surgical procedure, it is paramount that the nurse also give considerable thought to her role in assisting the anesthesiologist or nurse anesthetist. Again, a cooperative team effort is involved in the care of the dependent patient, and the anesthesiologist plays a vital role. The patient must not be subjected to more anesthesia than is absolutely necessary, since it is an unnatural state. Therefore, all delays that would unnecessarily prolong anesthesia time should be kept to a minimum.

The OR must be in perfect readiness for the patient. Just as you must assure that the equipment is present and in working order for the surgeon, and that the table parts (stirrups, braces, etc.) are ready for positioning the patient, so you must assure that the equipment is present for the anesthesiologist. That does not simply mean assuring that the anesthesia machine is in the room—it refers to IV poles, arm boards, monitors, working suction, etc. *For example:*

1. Reading the chart in advance reveals information about the *individual* patient—and *individual* needs.

2. Conferring with the anesthesiologist before surgery alerts the nurse to the patient's specific anesthesia requirements.

3. Evaluating the room setup before the patient enters (using the Mental Lineup) will confirm the presence of basic needs.

Those efforts prevent last-minute scurrying by the circulating nurse to obtain supplies, which would consequently necessitate her absence from the room, and especially from the patient.

Anesthesiologists usually have special apparatus and needed supplies at their fingertips, but they depend upon the nurse to see that the anesthesia stands are correctly supplied (e.g., with syringes, ECG pads, airways, endotracheal tubes, IV solutions, breathing circuits). It is the nurse's responsibility to:

1. Be sure supplies are replaced between operations.

2. Provide the anesthesiologist with an area for placement of used supplies. It facilitates collection and removal from the room.

3. Provide a receptacle for syringes and needle wrappers, or other such method as is used for inventory.

4. Be sure that suction apparatus is in working order.

a. A small basin of water may be required to clean suction of tenacious material.
b. All tubing and connections must be immediately available.
c. Deep tracheal suction requires sterile catheter technique.

QUIET ENVIRONMENT

There are several opinions as to whether the patient hears or remembers conversation during anesthesia. Therefore, some thoughts are worth consideration:

1. Patients have reported and repeated conversations heard during operative procedures—when it was assumed they were "asleep." Therefore, conversations during surgery should be restrained, whether or not references are made to the patient or to extraneous subjects.

2. A patient may be unduly apprehensive and alarmed, or may be hyperactive at the time of induction. Thus, some feel that softly spoken, encouraging words and explanations (e.g., "You will begin to feel sleepy; you are all right") reassure the patient as he is going to sleep, with the result that he will awaken with the same assurance.

3. All feel that external stimuli can destroy the effects of the preoperative medication and cause a "stormy induction."

In any event, it is important that nurses be aware that the surgical patient experiences an emotional trauma, whether he receives a general, regional, or local anesthetic.

RESTRAINING A PATIENT

Evaluate your patient in terms of size, age, emotional state, effect of preliminary medication, and disease condition. Remember that you restrain a patient to protect him from injuring himself (by falling, dislodging an intravenous, accidentally putting his hand in the wound, or contaminating the sterile drapes).

Be aware that some people have a phobia toward restraints. They become very apprehensive if restraints are put in place when they are awake. Hence, your words of assurance and your actions must be geared toward attempting to overcome the patient's fears. Below are various forms of restraint used in some operating rooms, and their indications for use.

Leg strap. Check with the OR policy to ascertain if it is routine procedure to place a leg strap before induction of anesthesia, after induction, or if it is used at all. The leg strap is usually placed above the knees, allowing room for the thickness of your hand, in order not to restrict circulation. Be sure to explain to the patient, if he is awake, what you are doing. For example, you might say, "Because the OR bed is narrow, I am placing a strap—like a seat belt—to make you feel more secure."

Note: Years ago, the primary purpose of the strap was to literally hold down the patient when he became active during the excitement stage of anesthesia. Today, modern anesthesia methods and newer drugs may reduce or eliminate the excitement period, but it still may occur.

Wristlets. If they are applied when the patient is awake, explain what you are doing. But whether the patient is awake or asleep, be sure his hands and arms are in a natural anatomical position, and that they are correctly supported and padded for comfort and protection from table parts.

Emotional restraint. Be aware that just your presence is comforting to the patient. This "emotional restraint" can make the use of physical measures unnecessary. For example, in the case of a child who is undergoing anesthesia:

1. The preoperative medication and a quiet room may make the child unaware of, or easily submissive to, the introduction of inhalation gases.

2. The circulating nurse can distract the alert child by talking about pleasant activities, singing a song with him, etc. In any event, the nurse must be prepared to keep the child from suddenly moving about the OR bed, grabbing the mask or tubing, or falling.

3. Discuss with your supervisor the methods employed at your hospital.

4. Be aware that gentle holding (not forcible restraint) of the arms around the wrist area, and guidance (rather than restraint) of movements are advisable.

TYPES OF ANESTHESIA

Listed below are the various types of anesthesia used in the OR, and their definitions.

Local. Infiltration into the general area of operation, without selecting a specific nerve to anesthetize, e.g., injection of lidocaine around the area of the nevus that is to be removed.

Topical.   A properly buffered solution applied to a surface (skin or mucous membrane), e.g., the anesthesiologist may spray the vocal cords and larynx with lidocaine before inserting the endotracheal tube.

Regional nerve block.   Injection of solution of proper dilution into tissue in the immediate proximity of the regional nerve itself, e.g., a brachial block for upper extremity surgery.

Caudal and *epidural.*   Injection of anesthetic drug of proper dilution into the caudal or epidural space, bathing the nerves that supply the area in which the procedure is to take place. (There are fewer side effects than with spinal anesthesia.) These types of regional anesthesia can be used for more extensive operations than can a regional nerve block, e.g., hemorrhoidectomy, herniorrhaphy, vaginal delivery, hysterectomy.

Spinal.   Injection of drug of proper dilution into the subdural space, where it mixes with cerebrospinal fluid, bathing the nerves in the subdural (subarachnoid) space.

General anesthesia.   The rendering of the patient into an unconscious state and insensible to pain, which can be done by intravenous, inhalation, or a combination of agents.

Note: At one time it was necessary to induce "deep" anesthesia to obtain the necessary condition for surgical procedures. Now, with the use of IV drugs, which relax the muscles (often referred to as "muscle relaxants"), a proper condition can be obtained without "deep" anesthesia. However, the anesthesiologist must maintain adequate ventilation, either manually or with an anesthesia ventilator.

Again, be aware that even though the patient may appear to be sleeping, he may well be aware of the environment.

BASIC CONSIDERATIONS

Basic considerations as to the care of the patient undergoing anesthesia are these:

1. Be aware that induction of the patient and the patient's emergence from anesthesia are crucial times for the patient (vomiting most often occurs at those times).

2. The scrub nurse (or scrub assistant) should be gowned and gloved in readiness for an emergent procedure, as well as for the surgeon's entrance.

3. The circulating nurse must be free to stay with the patient. (How can she do that if she has to tie your gown or open a pack?)

4. Await the anesthesiologist's permission before touching the patient or exposing the area for skin preparation. In engaging in such actions:
   a. You may upset the course of induction and evoke unwanted reflexes, such as laryngospasm.
   b. You may cause the patient to move and disrupt positioning or contaminate a sterile area.

5. During injection of medication for local anesthesia:
   a. Observe the patient for adverse reaction.
   b. Anticipate the possible need for medication to counteract toxic reaction. (Some feel it advisable to have a syringe of Pentothal in readiness.)

c. Although policies of the OR vary as to care of patients undergoing local anesthesia, it is agreed that they should be monitored. Individual practices, such as routine use of electrocardiogram monitors or automatic blood pressure machines, or whether such patients should have IVs started, are usually OR ground rules for safe practice.

6. Determine the nurse power and equipment needed during regional anesthesia. *For example:*
   a. The circulating nurse has to pour prep solution and perhaps supply the anesthesiologist with needles or anesthetic solution.
   b. Caudal anesthesia for hemorrhoidectomy may require you to flex the table and provide additional arm boards for a comfortable position.
   c. A spinal or epidural may be administered with the patient in a sitting position. Have a stool ready to support the patient's feet. A spinal or epidural can be given with the patient lying on his side, and the nurse holding him in a position so that his back is arched.

   Additional nurse power may be needed to quickly change the patient's position for surgery to prevent spread of the anesthetic drug.

7. When no anesthesia is required (e.g., in some hospitals certain examinations and cast changes are done in the OR), be sure that assistance can be summoned quickly in the event of sudden untoward patient reaction.

8. Be aware that acute emergency patients are perhaps the most poorly prepared for anesthesia. *For example:*

    a. Such patients may have just eaten or taken liquids (aspiration possibility). Following traumatic injury or the start of labor, the stomach does not empty in the normal time, often retaining its contents.

    b. The patient may have been in poor health before the accident and a history may be unattainable.

    c. The patient may be intoxicated or, because of head injury, may be semicomatose, but very agitated; his medical history may be unavailable (he may be unable to communicate, and no relative can be reached). Thus, there is the possibility of presence of cardiac or respiratory ailment, which is unknown at time of surgery.

9. Be observant and apply your nursing knowledge.

    a. Anticipate the anesthesiologist's requests—know the usual procedure and observe the patient.

    b. Know the location of the "crash cart," the procedure for alerting the control desk to difficulties, and the OR procedure for conducting a "code" situation.

10. Do not use the anesthesiologist's table or machine for placement of your supplies:

    a. It encumbers his work.

    b. It prevents quick access to his supplies.

11. If sprays (e.g., adhesives, benzoin) are used at the operative field, exercise caution. *For example:*

    a. Protect the patient from inadvertent inhalation of sprays.

    b. Protect the patient's eyes from inadvertent contact with sprays.

    c. Protect apparatus from gummy materials.

12. Confirm with the anesthesiologist the name and type of anesthesia administered, before recording it on the operative record.

13. At the end of the operation:
    a. Remain with the patient and anesthesiologist.
    b. Be aware of intravenous containers, tubing, and injection sites, and prevent accidental dislodgment, breakage, etc.
    c. Move the patient gently (when the anesthesiologist gives permission).

KNOW HOW TO CARE FOR
ANESTHESIA EQUIPMENT

Today, most of the anesthesia supplies are disposable. However, some items are nondisposable. You should know the difference, and the physical properties of each—as you may be requested to care for them. *For example:*

1. Certain equipment cannot withstand the high temperatures of steam sterilizers.

2. If ethylene oxide sterilization is to be used, be aware that an adequate aeration process is necessary.

3. If a disinfecting solution is used, be sure it will not cause skin irritation (certain porous materials absorb the solution). Check the disinfectant preferred. Be sure the article is *thoroughly* rinsed and dried.

4. Machines, tanks, etc., must be clean before they are moved into the OR.
    a. Certain companies supply small tanks in plastic wrap to minimize dust during transport (remove

the cover when you are outside the OR). Wipe off other types of tanks with a water-dampened cloth.

b. Do not attempt to clean a machine without knowing proper instructions. Certain solutions can cause corrosion. Oils must not be used (they can combine with the oxygen under pressure and cause fire).

5. If requested to open the sterile anesthesia procedural tray, exercise optimum sterile technique.

The policies of the specific OR determine who moves the anesthesia machines between cases (if it is necessary), and who connects the machines to the gas supply. Do not move a machine unless you are properly instructed. Listed below are general guidelines for care of anesthesia machines.

1. Improper pressure on regulators, valves, gauges, etc., causes dislodgement, gas leaks, costly repairs, and injuries. Tightening valves excessively may break delicate parts.

2. Proper handling by the rail handles on the machine prevents damage.

3. Anesthesia machines should be moved slowly and carefully, so that they will not tip over, and in order to prevent canisters or protruding parts from striking doors, etc.

4. Note the color coding of gas lines, and be aware that machines are "pin indexed." (This means that each gas type has a different connector to the machine, which prevents potential errors in administering the incorrect agent.)

Note: It is incumbent upon the individual anesthesi-
       ologist to check his equipment and make sure it
       is functioning properly.

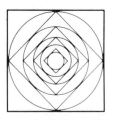

Chapter 18

Admission of the Patient to the Operating Room Suite

The patient awaiting surgery undergoes great emotional stress. A person in apparent good health, who requires a very minor operative procedure, may be as mentally distressed as one seriously ill who is about to undergo lengthy major surgery.

Proper identification of the patient at all times is of paramount importance. This is a responsibility that cannot be overemphasized, and it is the responsibility of each member of the staff who has any contact with the patient.

ARRIVAL OF THE PATIENT
IN THE OPERATING ROOM SUITE

The nurse receiving the patient should introduce herself, and ask the patient both his name and his surgeon's name. She should then check the identification bracelet, as well as the name on the chart. Doing so:

1. Helps the nurse regard the patient as a person instead of a procedure.

2. Reassures the patient—he sees that personal interest is taken.

3. Acts as a first check in establishing the identity of the patient and its correlation with the name band and chart name.

4. Gives the nurse an opportunity, through the initial meeting, to note any untoward factors of the patient's condition that should be reported to the surgeon and the anesthesiologist.

The charge nurse should check the chart and the patient as follows:

1. Check the name on the chart with the name on the operative schedule.

2. Check the correlation of the surgeon's name and diagnosis with that of the operative schedule.

3. Check the patient's name on the identification band or name tag secured to the patient.

4. Check for the presence of an operative permit (signed, dated, and witnessed). It is imperative that the hospital rules regarding operative permits be carried out. Hospitals vary in their requirements, but all permits are designed to protect the patient, the doctors and nurses, and the hospital. Some considerations are:
   a. The patient should write his name in full (avoid

initials). In the case of a married woman, her first name (e.g., Mary Doe) should be given, not her husband's name (e.g., Mrs. John Doe).

b. A minor (under the age of 18) must have the signature of a parent or guardian. A minor who is married or earning his own living is considered an emancipated minor, and his signature is usually sufficient. Check your hospital policy for variances.

c. If the patient cannot write and makes his mark (e.g., "X"), it is safe practice to have it followed by the statement "his mark," and a witnessing signature.

d. If the patient is unconscious and his family unavailable, obey hospital policy.

e. Telephone consents are not safe practice, but there are emergent situations when a consent is obtained via telephone (e.g., from a relative of a patient not capable of giving consent, but who requires immediate treatment). The surgeon's conversation with the party, and the party's consent, is listened to by a witness (often a nurse). The surgeon writes a descriptive statement of the conversation, and both he and the witness sign the statement (also noting the date and hour).

f. A signature written as consent after the preliminary medication is given may be considered invalid, as the patient under narcosis is not responsible for his actions. Check your hospital and state rules for the legality of consents.

g. The operative permit also states the proposed surgery. Read it carefully and correlate it with the operative schedule; note in particular the words "right" or "left," and confirm the surgery and operative side with the patient.

5. Check the time of administration and dosage of preliminary medication. It is important information for the anesthesiologist.

6. Check the recording of the history and physical examination (including normal blood pressure), and check for any reported allergies. It is important information for the surgeon, the anesthesiologist, and the nurses in the post-anesthesia room.

7. Check to see if reports on laboratory work are present. The surgeon and anesthesiologist will want to know if urine tests show albumin, acetone, or sugar. They will also want to know the results of blood tests. If hemoglobin is below 10 grams, oxygen transport is lessened, as is reserve for potential surgical blood loss.

8. Check for dentures, jewelry, artificial parts, etc., and remove them for the patient's safety (they must be signed for and taken care of per hospital policy).

Note: Today, the use of contact lenses is common. Be aware that lenses are not easily seen and are hazardous to the unconscious patient.

9. Check for the presence of eye makeup. It can cause irritation to the delicate eye structure, should it enter the eye accidentally.

10. Check the prepared operative area. It must:
    a. Conform to the surgeon's orders.
    b. Be completed before the patient enters the specific operating room.

11. If all "checks" are correct and complete, re-identify the patient (and name band), and write the specific assigned OR number on the stretcher. (Be sure to underline the number in order to prevent confusion between numbers, e.g., 6 and 9.) Such a procedure:
    a. Prevents the patient from being transferred to the wrong room.
    b. Indicates that the chart has been checked, everything is in order, and the patient can be released from the waiting area.
12. If the chart information is not complete and the information shows deviation from the norm, the patient should not be transferred to the surgical room, for the following reasons:
    a. It may require contact with the nursing unit, the surgeon, or the laboratory for information.
    b. It may require cancellation of the case.
    c. It is done for the protection of the patient, the surgeon, and the hospital.

13. The charge nurse also notes the surgeon's requests (e.g., X-rays are present, radiology or pathology department is alerted, blood requests and blood availability are confirmed).

AWAITING TRANSFER TO SPECIFIC OPERATING ROOM
Do not leave the patient unattended.

1. The medicated patient is not responsible. (*Caution*: The patient who arrives quietly in the operating room may be the one who falls off the stretcher. Why? The noisy, restless patient will obviously not be left alone, but the quiet, sleepy patient is apt to

be. He may awake, forget he is on a stretcher, turn on his side, and fall to the floor.)

2. Intravenous treatments must be checked.

3. The presence of the nurse lends reassurance to the patient.

4. Untoward reactions may be noted and must be reported.

Minimize external stimuli.

1. Restrict conversation of staff.
   a. Conversation concerning the patient increases his anxiety.
   b. Conversation about personal matters reduces the patient's security.

2. Eliminate any unnecessary noise and activity. Such behavior:
   a. Stimulates the patient, thus reducing the effect of the preoperative medication.
   b. Tends to promote an atmosphere of confusion in the operating room.

TRANSFER TO
SPECIFIC OPERATING ROOM

The operating room must be in readiness. Doing so:

1. Eliminates confusion.

2. Ensures that the circulating nurse is free to care for the patient.

Recheck of the *chart* and *patient* is done by the circulating nurse as follows:

1. Patient's name (compare the name on the chart and identification band with the name of the patient scheduled for that room).

2. Diagnosis (check especially indication of *right* or *left* in cases of limbs, hernias, kidneys, breasts, etc. Do not rely on a prepped area to be the area of surgery).

3. Name of the surgeon in attendance (there may be more than one hernia operation going on in the operating room suite).

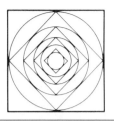

Chapter 19
Documentation

Throughout the book, reference is made to the documentation of facts and actions (e.g., recording of specimens, written verification of correct counts). Malpractice suits are not uncommon (unfortunately), and the hospital, the physician, and/or you can be the defendant(s). Proper documentation, therefore, is of prime importance.

The very patient charts are documentation of the patient's treatment, history, and facts. They not only serve as written proof of what has been done, but also may indicate the next step in the course of treatment. Consequently, the OR nurse must make sure that her charting is verifiable and complete. There are many medicolegal purposes of charting. *For example:*

1. A patient arrives in the OR, and is observed to have a bruise on the left forearm. Ask the patient how it happened and when. Record on the chart your observation and what the patient "states" (include the time of observation). *Purpose:*
   a. It verifies the incident did not occur in the OR.
   b. It alerts the next nurse for need of care.

2. Wound drains are inserted and anchored in place. Record the type of drain inserted and how many were used. *Purpose:*
   a. It is a safety factor for the patient.
   b. The next receiving nurse will be alerted to the care of dressings and potential drainage.
   c. The doctor is reminded of how many drains will have to be removed.

3. A patient arrives in the OR with jewelry or dentures. Assure safe care of the article, and call the nursing unit to retrieve it. Document and sign the chart (in the unit person's presence), indicating that the article (name and how many) was given to the person (write the person's name). Record the hour. In your presence, have the person sign a written statement, indicating that the article was received. *Purpose:*
   a. The nursing unit accepts responsibility for the article.
   b. The article is safely secured for the patient.

UNUSUAL INCIDENCES

An unusual incidence could be an inadvertent occurrence, or any injury to an employee or a patient. Hospitals require documentation of such events, and expect the OR nurse to comply with the hospital policy and procedure. Documentation is usually followed by some action. Basic considerations are:

1. The incident and action taken should be reported immediately.

2. The appropriate form must be completely filled out, and charting done, if required.

Note: The medicolegal point of view is that documentation of the incident indicates the occurrence or problem was recognized, and that steps were taken to remedy the situation. Ignoring or attempting to hide an incident compounds the problem, and is subject to legal complications.

Ask your supervisor for an explanation of what is considered an unusual incident and of the procedure to be followed.

CARE DOCUMENTATION FORMS

Most ORs provide specific documentation forms. *For example:*

1. An OR chart form (often referred to as an "OR Patient Diary"), which, upon completion, becomes a part of the chart.

2. A separate form for the legal OR register. This can be a permanent form retained by the OR, or an information form that is re-recorded in an OR register or put into a computer.

Note: If the OR does not have a specific OR diary, check with your supervisor as to what must be recorded and documented on the patient's chart.

PATIENT CHARGE DOCUMENTATION

Logically, the OR must charge the patient for services rendered. Each OR has established a method of patient charge and a format for listing the chargeable services. OR time, equipment (e.g., prosthesis, catheter), and drugs are some of the things for which the hospital must recoup compensation. To prevent lost charges, you must:

1. Investigate the billing method.

2. Know what items are chargeable.

3. Confirm the accurate recording (documentation) of what was used on the patient.

   Obviously, the patient must *not* be charged for something that was not used, and must not be responsible for the cost of a supply item that was wasted by the staff (e.g., the wrong size embolectomy catheter was opened and not used). It is also obvious that the hospital cannot economically withstand *lost charges* (e.g., an embolectomy catheter that was used and not recorded on the charge ticket).

QUALITY ASSURANCE

Surveying and accrediting agencies are very interested in the documentation of things that are indicative of *optimum quality care* of and for the patient. The purpose of such documentation is to assure the patient and the community that the hospital is safe, and identifies and rectifies problems, and that the environment, hospital practices, etc., promote the proper delivery of health care. *For example:*

1. The assurance of such quality is obtained by documented records by all hospital services.

2. The OR department is required to document the safe standards, policies, and procedures.

3. The OR staff must uphold these standards and document that they are practiced.

A few examples of quality assurance are:

1. The OR uses biological monitors to assure sterility of autoclaved supplies (instruments).
   a. Do you understand how spore tests are done? Where they are documented?
   b. Do you change the sterilizer graph daily? Record the date and sterilizer number? Save the graph for documentation?

2. The OR has educational standards, in-service sessions, etc., with skill-competency checklists.
   a. Do you keep lists up-to-date and provide written documentation?
   b. Do you request and attend in-service sessions when your knowledge of equipment is vague?

3. The OR maintains quality assurance with regard to drugs and narcotics records.
   a. Do you accurately chart medications?
   b. Do you confirm the narcotics count with another nurse and document by signatures?

SUMMARY

It is vital for you to follow the hospital regulations for documentation. Review the regulations, and do an advance review of any charting or special forms. And don't hesitate to ask questions when uncommon incidences or circumstances arise. Then, when recording information:

1. Confirm that all information is complete and legible, and contains the date, time, and appropriate signatures.

2. Safeguard the preservation of documentations

(e.g., see that they are placed in the chart or at the designated OR collection area).

Be aware that legal actions (malpractice suits) are not only instituted against the hospital and physician, but also against the nurse. You are responsible for your actions, and they must be supported by appropriate documentation.

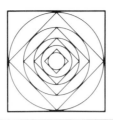

Chapter 20
Individualizing Patient Care

It has been mentioned before that there is no routine operation, just as there is no "routine" patient. Each patient scheduled for surgery is different, with different physical, psychological, and spiritual needs. For those reasons, keep the following points in mind:

1. Operating room personnel must realize that the patient in surgery participates in a preoperative as well as a postoperative phase of treatment that is closely connected to surgical intervention. The patient's individual makeup and the events that take place prior to surgery will affect his treatment in the operating room, and his postoperative treatment as well. Nurses and assistants on the patient units (floors) must also understand that surgery is closely allied to pre- and postoperative care.

2. Operating room and patient unit nursing personnel must realize that effective care is achieved through

close communication, the sharing of knowledge, and a joint team effort.

3. Preoperative, intraoperative, and postoperative care of the patient are now described as "perioperative nursing."

   a. The scope of the perioperative role can be broad, e.g., nursing unit/operating room/recovery room/nursing unit.

   b. The scope is also narrow. The OR nurse does perioperative nursing within the OR. The patient enters the suite (preoperative), has surgery (intra-operative), and is transferred to the recovery room unit (postoperative).

   c. This chapter's discussion promoting individualized patient care and continuity of care reinforces the perioperative care principle.

To hear a floor nurse say "Good luck!" to a patient going to surgery, as if he were entering the realm of chance, is very distressing. It is equally distressing, in another way, to see an operating room nurse deliver a patient to the post-anesthesia room without communicating information about his condition, or indicating the presence of drains or catheters, the type of surgical intervention, or such factors as "the patient is deaf."

In a sense, the operating room professional nurse and nursing assistant see the beginnings of individualized care when they select instruments, sutures, and the basic requirements for the specific operative procedure. The points listed throughout this book for the purpose of encouraging logical forethought also apply to the development of an individualized care plan. What is needed is a plan that is tailored to *Mr. Jones*, rather than to a cholecystectomy—a realistic plan that can be followed by the operating room nurse in difficult situations, as well as by the nurse in a well-staffed, not-too-busy OR.

There is much controversy as to whether the OR nurse must visit the patient preoperatively in order to meet his needs, or whether the floor nurse should witness the surgery in order to better plan for the patient's individual postoperative care. One point to bear in mind is this: If you cannot give that attention to *each* patient, then it is hardly fair or professional to single out a few. Nurses dedicated to good patient care, and who would really like to make both visits, are faced with the problem of unavailable time and staffing shortages. However, difficult conditions do not negate *your responsibility to render individualized care for each patient.*

To review:

1. Patient care begins the moment a person enters the hospital. He is the center and objective of the hospital organizational chart, regardless of his color, race, creed, or station in life; regardless of whether he is a friend or relative of someone on the staff, or whether circumstances forced his admission at other than the "routine hours."

2. A plan for meeting the patient's individual needs must not be solely dependent upon a preoperative visit by the OR nurse, nor must it wait until the floor (unit) nurse provides a written plan of care.

If we consider the patient's entire hospital stay as a continuous chain of events, all interrelated, two objectives for the operating room nurse become clear:

1. She must view surgery as a part of the "chain" and must see that continuity into the next area of care is maintained.

2. She must have a realistic method of individualizing care that:
   a. will apply to the first, second, and "nth" patient on the schedule;
   b. will apply to the emergency patient, regardless of when he is admitted or at what hour his surgery is to be performed; and
   c. will still be valid even in a case of the unpredicted absence of a particular staff member (who may have visited the patient preoperatively).

FACTORS IN AN INDIVIDUALIZED OR CARE PLAN

The following are necessary requirements for an effective individualized OR care plan:

1. *Communication.* Communication may take place at different times, for example, when the patient is scheduled, or when the surgeon or the anesthesiologist arrives on the unit. It continues to be possible when the patient is greeted in the OR suite. Communication entails the exchange of information between patient/nurses, family/nurses, surgeons and anesthesiologists/nurses, and nurses/nurses. It is either verbal or written, usually a combination of both. It may be telephoned, spoken face to face, or written on the chart.

2. *Coordination.* The registered professional nurse member of the room team is the nursing team leader; the OR charge nurse (if present) may be an

intermediary; the co-worker RN or surgical technologist of the room team is an active participant in the team conference and in treatment. All must work together.

3. *Categorizing.* The three main needs of the patient are physical, psychological, and spiritual. You may wish to subdivide these categories into others in order to enrich the plan, e.g., you may want to include safeguarding the patient as a special point.

LOGICAL THOUGHT AND ACTIVITY NECESSARY TO FORMULATE A PLAN

If you were asked to briefly describe the sequence of events that affect a surgical patient (without detail), you might state: "The case is booked; the nursing team prepares the setup, applying a Mental Lineup and Four-Clue System; the anesthesiologist arrives and prepares his equipment; the surgeon arrives and prepares to scrub; the patient unit is called, and the patient is brought to surgery, where he is greeted, admitted to the suite, and identified; the chart is reviewed; the surgical procedure is performed; and the patient is transferred to the post-anesthesia room."

The following is a list of those events, with some examples of individual needs and actions that can be taken to meet those needs. The examples are not complete in detail; so as you read each one, ask yourself "What else might be added?" and "What other actions might be taken?"

Topic 1. Pertinent information obtained at the time of scheduling. This will include the patient's name, surgical procedure, etc.; however, you should also record in the "remarks" column pertinent descriptions and special requests, such as "cardiac," "obese," "blind"; "will need Prolene mesh" (or cautery, or X-ray).

Action: Consider need for monitor; determine number of personnel and degree of experience needed for the patient assignment. Remember that additional verbal support and personal contact will be needed for the blind person. Are Prolene mesh and cautery available? (What else might you add?)

Topic 2. Team leader confers with the nursing team. The *first* aspect is preparing for *physical care*.

Action: Review the points of the Mental Lineup and Four-Clue System; see that the pattern is set up to meet the needs of the patient that were established at the time of booking. Be prepared to take care of other special needs that will be communicated later.

The *second* aspect is preparing to meet the *psychological needs* of the patient. His self-esteem must be preserved, for he is now in a dependent role. You may assume, whether evident or not, that the patient is apprehensive and needs emotional support.

Action: Refer to Chapters 2 and 18.

The *third* aspect is preparing to meet the *spiritual needs* of the patient.

Action: Alert the patient unit, if the operative time has been changed. Perhaps the patient has arranged for a visit from a member of the clergy. Missing the clergyman because of advancement in schedule will further upset the patient. If the patient arrives wearing a religious medal, prevent its loss. In the event of unexpected death, note the patient's religion, and follow institutional policy.

Topic 3. Conference with the anesthesiologist. This will communicate what the anesthesiologist has observed in his visit, e.g., the size of the patient, respiratory problems, or extreme apprehension; and what his specific requests are for induction of the patient.

Action: Use forethought to obtain the necessary supplies, drugs, and additional nurse power, and to provide psychological support.

Topic 4.   Conference with the surgeon.   This may reveal a deviation in his surgical approach, or may uncover anticipated problems, e.g., the patient has been operated on before, or the surgeon would like a size 16 Foley catheter inserted.

Action: Organize positioning plan; discuss operative approach with scrub nurse; obtain appropriate catheterization set and catheter.

Topic 5.   Conference with the nurse of the patient unit.   This may reveal that the patient has an intravenous running, or that the patient has stated he is allergic to adhesive tape.

Action: Have the IV pole in readiness; observe the injection site, type of fluid, and any reactions; obtain nonallergenic tape for the surgical dressing and for the anesthesiologist's use.

Topic 6.   Provisions for safeguarding the patient.

Action: Identify the patient; check the chart for special details (see Chapter 18) and for written notes concerning *this* patient. Follow rules to prevent infection, to assure proper positioning, etc.

Topic 7.   Communication with the patient.   This allows for visual observation and evaluation, as well as verbal contact, e.g., the patient states his mouth is dry, or suddenly feels tightness in his chest, or you observe a tearful expression.

Action: Moisten patient's lips with wet gauze; explain that the medication is causing the dryness; report chest pain to surgeon and anesthesiologist; allay fears and give emotional support.

Topic 8.   Assist the surgical team and provide for continuous care.

Action: Do necessary charting; care for specimens and cultures properly. Inform next unit of special needs, e.g., oxygen, respirator, heating or cooling blankets. Communicate to receiving nurse the type of operation, presence of catheters, etc.

You can see how such information demonstrates that each patient is a person, not just a surgical procedure. You can also see that you are using the nursing process of assessment, planning, implementation, and evaluation.

Table 20-1 is an example of an individualized care plan employed for an emergency in the late evening hours, when there is no time to visit the patient. Even here, determining the need for "prompt action" does not require "technical" skill, but rather good, basic nursing technique, and use of the nursing process. *Organized thought, logical reasoning,* and *good communication* are employed.

Even though the operating room is different from a nursing unit, and one hospital will be different from another, the goal of total care remains. Use the framework presented in Table 20-1, and alter it to meet the requirements of your particular institution.

It is suggested that the new operating room nurse or surgical technologist choose a patient and procedure at random, and prepare a care plan. Write it down if necessary. In doing this, the nurse develops the ability to review the topics mentally (*without* writing), and when called upon to apply the various elements of each patient's plan, she can do so in quick succession.

Table 20-1

EXAMPLE OF AN INDIVIDUALIZED CARE PLAN

Emergency Bronchoscopy for Removal of Foreign Body

Topic	Action
1. Pertinent information obtained when scheduled	
Name of patient, unit location	Assure accurate spelling.
What is foreign body—Pin? Coin? Bone?	Visualize type of grasper and setup that will be needed.
Patient is 7 years old.	Select child-size equipment.
2. Team conference concerning:	
Physical needs	
Foreign body to be removed via bronchoscope; special positioning and setup	Apply Mental Lineup and Four-Clue System; have oxygen and suction apparatus ready.
Will need recovery room care	Notify recovery room of case.
Psychological needs	
Child will have to leave parents.	Be understanding and empathetic.
Child is frightened of strange surroundings; is hyperactive.	Stay with child; comfort him; offer assurance.
Spiritual needs (This aspect will probably be attended to in the emergency room.)	Offer comfort; apply the best patient care you can, as if the patient were your own child.

Continued

Table 20-1 *continued*

Topic	Action
3. Conference with anesthesiologist Patient has just had full meal; is crying and restless.	Ensure that suction apparatus is in working order (see Chapter 16 re induction of children).
4. Conference with surgeon History and physical examination show draining infected area on leg. After bronchoscopy, surgeon desires to culture and dress area.	Prepare and exercise proper techniques; have culture equipment and dressing set ready.
5. Conference with emergency room charge nurse Patient's nickname is "Skippy." Preop urine specimen could not be obtained. Parents will be waiting in lobby.	Use nickname when talking to child. Be sure surgeon and anesthesiologist are informed. Make written note of message for surgeon.
6. Safeguard patient (additional physical need) Child cannot be depended upon to say proper name. Patient's chart in order (consent of parents, history and physical, etc.) Child is restless on stretcher.	Check identification band, chart, etc. (see Chapter 18). Surgeon may proceed. Stay with child.

7. Communication with patient

Child is crying for his mother.	Use child's nickname; assure him his mother is waiting for him.
Child seems uncooperative; is waving arms about.	Be patient; guide his motions to prevent injury to himself.

8. Assist surgical team and provide for continuous care

Patient anesthetized; foreign particle removed	Assist in performance of surgical team; provide care of specimen.
Culture taken; leg area dressed	Assure care of culture; do necessary charting.
Patient transferred to recovery area	Provide proper stretcher, side rails, nurse attendance.

Communication with recovery room nurse

Special information given to nurse (verbal and written)	Relate the following information: procedure done, presence of infected area on leg, ingestion of food a short time ago, patient's nickname, need of urine specimen; assist nurse if necessary.
Parents very anxious	Surgeon knows parents are waiting in lobby; he will notify them when they can see their child.

PREOPERATIVE PATIENT VISIT

As mentioned earlier, the preoperative patient visit depends upon the hospital policy, kinds of training programs, and objectives of nursing service. It can be advantageous both for the patient and the nurse, when used properly. An effective visit must have a particular purpose, and that purpose must be understood. Principles of an effective preoperative patient visit are:

1. Know what information you are allowed to give, and what purpose your visit is to serve (e.g., meeting the patient, allaying his fears of the unknown, skin preparation, individual needs).

2. Be sure you are not asking the patient questions that he has already been asked. It is annoying to the patient.

3. Exchange information with the unit nurse, and review patient data and the preoperative checklist.

4. Have a professional demeanor, and be sure your personal appearance is acceptable.

5. Hold a conference with your supervisor and other OR personnel concerning your observations and results of the visit.

POSTOPERATIVE PATIENT VISIT

The principles discussed above concerning the preoperative patient visit are applicable to the postoperative patient visit as well.

If the practice cannot be carried out consistently, there is an alternative that can be used at least once for each member of the OR nursing team, that is, to accompany a surgeon when he makes surgical "rounds" (most surgeons are happy to cooperate). Again, the activity must have a clearly understood purpose. Results of the postoperative patient visit are:

1. It reinforces the individuality of each patient for the nurse.

2. The nurse sees the continuity of patient care.

3. Such visits make clear the results of surgical intervention and the progress of the patient.

4. Postoperative visits provide subject matter for operating room conferences.

Individualizing patient care is an entire team effort, as is a surgical procedure, achieved through logical forethought and action.

Appendix

Surgical Terminology

The nurse who is new to operating room procedures is rather suddenly exposed to surgical nomenclature. It is essential that she understand the terms used, in order to interpret the operative schedule, understand the patient's diagnosis, follow directions, and perform as an efficient member of the surgical team.

There are no shortcuts for learning the vocabulary of any language. Constant attention to classroom instruction, frequent use of references, and study are requisites for intelligent action.

By examining a word for the root or common term, and then noting the prefix or suffix, you can usually determine its meaning. For example, if you were told that "-ectomy" meant "removal of," would it not be reasonable to say that *appendectomy* meant *removal of the appendix?* Applying that knowledge, you could then deduce that *tonsillectomy* meant *removal of the tonsil(s).* However, as the word *cyst* means bladder *or* sac, a *cystectomy* could mean either the removal of the urinary bladder or of another type of sac, such as a *cyst* of the arm. The latter example illustrates the need for careful interpretation of the operative schedule and an awareness of the interchangeability of word elements.

Table A-1 lists some prefixes, suffixes, and combining forms used in surgical terminology, together with their meanings. Whole-word examples derived from those elements are then provided.

Table A-1
PREFIXES, SUFFIXES, AND COMBINING FORMS USED IN SURGICAL TERMINOLOGY

Prefix/Suffix/ Combining Form	Meaning	Example
a-/an-	not, without	*a*septic
bi-	two, twice	*bi*lateral
-cele	hernia, swelling, tumor	recto*cele*
-cide	destructive	germi*cide*
cryo-	cold	*cryo*surgery
dis-	separation, negation, or reversal	*dis*infect
-ectomy	surgical removal of or cutting out	gastr*ectomy*
endo-	within	*endo*scopy
-esthesia	sensation	an*esthesia*
ex-	out of	*ex*cise
-gram	picture or tracing	cysto*gram*
hemi-	half	*hemi*colectomy
in-	in, into	*in*cision
-itis	inflammation	appendic*itis*
-lith/litho-	stone, calculus	chole*lith*/*litho*tomy
lysis/-lysis	destruction, a setting free	*lysis* of adhesions/ chemonucleo*lysis*
-(o)logy	study of	patho*logy*
-oma	tumor	carcin*oma*
-(o)rrhaphy	a suturing	hernio*rrhaphy*
-(o)scopy	inspection, looking into	cysto*scopy*
-(o)stomy	to furnish with an opening or outlet	gastro*stomy*
-(o)tomy	incision into	gastro*tomy*
pan-	entire, all	*pan*hysterectomy
-pexy	fixation	hystero*pexy*
-plasty	reconstruction or repair	rhino*plasty*

Prefix/Suffix/ Combining Form	Meaning	Example
-scope	(an instrument for) seeing or observing	cysto*scope*
septic-	pertaining to sepsis, infected	*septic*emia
supra-	above, excess	*supra*pubic
-tome	a cutting instrument	adeno*tome*
trauma-/ traumato	an injury or wound	*trauma*tize/ *traumato*pathy
-tripsy (trypsin)	crush or disintegrate	litho*tripsy*

Surgical terminology contains word roots that refer to a particular anatomical structure or body substance. Table A-2 gives such roots, indicates the body reference, and provides examples of words derived from both those roots and from suffixes listed in Table A-1.

Table A-2
WORD ROOTS USED IN SURGICAL TERMINOLOGY

Root	Body Reference	Example
blephar(o)-	eyelid	blepharoplasty
cardio-	heart	cardiotomy
cholecyst-	gallbladder	cholecystectomy
col-	colon	colectomy
derm(at)-	skin	dermatome
gastr(o)-	stomach	gastrostomy
gloss-	tongue	glossectomy
hem(at)-	blood	hemolysis
hepat(o)-	liver	hepatectomy
hyster(o)-	uterus	hysterectomy
nephr(o)-	kidney	nephrectomy
neur(o)-	nerve	neurorrhaphy
ophthalm(o)-	eye	ophthalmology

Continued

Table A-2 *continued*

Root	Body Reference	Example
orchid(o)-/orchi(o)-	testicle, testis	orchiectomy
osteo-	bone	osteotomy
oto-	ear	otoplasty
pneumo(n)-	lung	pneumonectomy
rhino-	nose	rhinoplasty

Practice is essential. Take time to review the operative schedule and to logically interpret the surgical terminology.

Epilogue

Operating room nursing provides a vital link in the chain of total patient care. The OR nurse must assure that the link is strong, and that the care of the patient is optimum.

There is a logic to OR nursing. The activities incorporate basic principles that can be logically applied to varying situations.

Set high goals for yourself, be a conscientious team member, and make learning an everyday process.

Other Titles of
Related Interest From
MEDICAL ECONOMICS BOOKS

Trauma Nursing
Edited by Virginia D. Cardona, RN, MS, CCRN
ISBN 0-87489-341-0

Shock: A Nursing Guide
Jacqueline M. Carolan, RN, BSN, CCRN
ISBN 0-87489-346-1

Managing the Critically Ill Effectively
Edited by Margaret Van Meter, RN
ISBN 0-87489-274-0

Critical Care Nursing Review and Self-Test
Billie C. Meador, RN, MSN, CCRN
ISBN 0-87489-300-3

Complete Guide to Cancer Nursing
Edited by Marjorie Beyers, RN, PhD,
Suzanne Durburg, RN, BSN, MEd, and
June Werner, RN, MSN, CNAA
ISBN 0-87489-294-5

Nurses' Guide to Neurosurgical Patient Care
Patricia Rauch Rhodes, RN, CNRN
ISBN 0-87489-223-6

**Pediatric Nursing Policies, Procedures,
and Personnel**
Eileen M. Sporing, RN, MSN,
Mary K. Walton, RN, MSN, and
Charlotte E. Cady, RN, MSN
ISBN 0-87489-339-9

Understanding Medications: The Hows and Whys of Drug Therapy
Morton J. Rodman, PhD
ISBN 0-87489-252-X

RN Medication Tips
Sara J. White, RPh, and
Karin Williamson, RN
ISBN 0-87489-251-1

Giving Medications Correctly and Safely
Andrew J. Bartilucci, PhD, and
Jane M. Durgin, CIJ, RN, MS
ISBN 0-87489-216-3

How to Calculate Drug Dosages
Angela R. Pecherer, RN, and
Suzanne L. Vertuno, RN
ISBN 0-87489-140-X

Drug Interactions Index
Fred Lerman, MD, and
Robert T. Weibert, PharmD
ISBN 0-87489-266-X

Manual for IV Therapy Procedures, Second Edition
Shila R. Channell, RN, MSN, PhD
ISBN 0-87489-370-4

A Guide to IV Admixture Compatibility, Third Edition
New England Deaconess Hospital, Boston
ISBN 0-87489-248-1

Manual of Operating Room Management
Jacqueline Willingham Cordner, RN, CNOR
ISBN 0-87489-260-0

RN Nursing Assessment Series

The Well Adult
ISBN 0-87489-281-3

Respiratory Problems
ISBN 0-87489-282-1

Metabolic Problems
ISBN 0-87489-284-8

Gastrointestinal Problems
ISBN 0-87489-285-6

Genitourinary Problems
ISBN 0-87489-286-4

Neurologic Problems
ISBN 0-87489-287-2

Musculoskeletal Problems
ISBN 0-87489-288-0

Cardiovascular Problems
ISBN 0-87489-289-9

The Well Infant and Child
ISBN 0-87489-290-2

RN's Survival Sourcebook: Coping With Stress
Gloria Ferraro Donnelly, RN, MSN
ISBN 0-87489-299-6

For information, write to:
MEDICAL ECONOMICS BOOKS
Oradell, New Jersey 07649
Or dial toll-free: 1-800-223-0581, ext. 2755
(Within the 201 area: 262-3030, ext. 2755)